FUK YU!

A Sweet and Sour Cancer Journey, Hong Kong Style

Hilary Faulkner

First Published in Hong Kong in 2019 by

Hilary Faulkner

Second Edition

Printed in Hong Kong by The Green Pagoda Press Ltd

The author of this book does not dispense medical advice or prescribe the use of any technique as a form of treatment for physical or medical problems without the advice of a physician. The intent of the author is only to offer information of a general nature that may help you keep well. In the event, you use any of the information in this book to treat yourself, which you are at liberty to do, the author assumes no responsibility for your actions.

The Poem 'A Mothers Love' is released with permission from Proverse Publishing Hong Kong; taken from 'Mingled Voices 3' Poetry Anthology 2019 Proverse International Poetry Competition – entry by Hilary Faulkner

ISBN: 978-988-74133-1-8

Facebook Page: A Sweet and Sour Cancer Journey, Hong Kong Style

e-mail: sweetandsourcancerjourney@gmail.com

www.sweetandsourcancerjourney.com

Dedication

Sadly, some of my fellow cancer thrivers are no longer with us today and completed their journey by gaining their angel wings. For me this is by far the hardest part.

This book is dedicated to them all, May You Rest In Peace my dear friends......................

Crane Tsuru Chen

Penny A

Liz V

Caroline R

Claire H

Stuart H

Dawn W

Alison H

Lesley D

Patricia S

Lisa H

Helene A

Susan G

Julie SJ

Julie S

Wendy L

PW & SJ

A Mothers Love

This unwanted canker grows inside me,
Taking over my body, slowly eating away,
Some say I should embrace it as my friend,
Accept it as part of me and nurture it,
On a good day this is my goal,
A presence within me to look after,
But when the headaches, the nausea,
The diarrhea, the fatigue, the hot sweats,
Take over, I cry, get out, go away,
Leave me alone, you are not my friend,
You are a cruel, nasty, enemy,
Ruining my life, I want to end it all.

Then I look towards my wonderful mum,
90 years old and seen so much in her life,
I am enfolded in her warm, loving arms,
She is my rock,
She is my confidante,
She keeps me going,
She understands and sees this horrible cancer journey first hand,
Without her love and support I would
Be living in such a dark place.
Every night before we sleep, we hug
As if it could be the last time,
Goodnight mum, Goodnight daughter,
Love you, sweet dreams............

Preface

I am writing this book to help all cancer thrivers on their journey of hope and to also help friends and family to understand the trials and tribulations of having this disease, whatever stage it might have been diagnosed.

In my case, ovarian cancer is often diagnosed too late, so I also hope that this book raises awareness of this specific cancer and helps any fellow sufferers.

The title of the book came from my feeling about this journey with an Asian twist as I am here in Hong Kong. I do feel like saying 'f*ck you cancer' and often my fellow cancer thrivers will say I'm having a 'f*ck it day today'. So, I hope the title isn't offensive and you have a chuckle at the pun. It has all definitely been very sweet and sour. The joy of making so many genuine lifelong friends is so sweet and the euphoria of having a good scan result, seeing drugs working! But the cancer itself, the treatments, the surgery, the stress of dealing with insurance companies, the scanxiety are definitely the sour part. Sadly, more sour than sweet but it is what it is.

My family are very private people so this is not an outpouring of how I feel emotionally on a more spiritual level or how I address my mortality. To be honest I haven't really thought about it in great detail but I know I will if I get to the stage when I can see that the cancer is beating me. I may be writing more about this journey as time goes on, (as it is just that, a lifelong journey); how my family reacted, or felt about things, or how I feel about them, with the exception of my mum who I mention several times in this book and who was 91 years old this year. This book is much more (I hope) a detailed support and guide for other cancer patients and their families embarking on this journey.

I am by no means a medical expert, this book is written from my point of view as a patient so it is not meant to give specific medical advice, but more to help the reader to ask questions and to think about the options they have. I may cause offence to some of the practitioners mentioned, but not by name, however this is the way I felt at the time and stand by my comments.

The book is a bit of a 'cathartic' download of my complete cancer journey, so without breaking up the story I have added an appendix at the back with clinical and drug information and other useful references, which I urge the reader to refer to.

Chapters

Sometimes ovarian cancer is whispering, please listen and don't ignore the symptoms!

Toilet habits, i.e. Urinating more frequently

Eating less and feeling full

Abdominal pain & bloating that persists

Lower back pressure & pain

Chapter One

The Journey Begins

My cancer journey, as I now call it, began very suddenly in March 2014. I was happily on my way to work on the ferry from Discovery Bay on the lovely island of Lantau where I was lucky enough to be living at that time, and suddenly felt something go pop inside. It was excruciatingly painful and I thought to myself 'something's not right here!' I immediately turned around and got the next ferry back and went in to see my doctor. He examined me and said it was in all likelihood a burst ovarian cyst. Being over 50 and post-menopausal I'd had these before and so was not too worried. He gave me a shot of Pethidine and told me to go home and sleep and if the pain didn't go away to come back.

It didn't go, so I returned the following day. He said 'We'd better send you for a scan then, just to see what's going on inside'. I'd felt no symptoms for anything else really, yes, a bit of backache, needing to urinate more often and a bit of bloating, but who doesn't get that over 50 when you are perhaps not as active and as fit as you could be!

I was referred for an external ultrasound, thank goodness not an internal one at this stage, as you always have to have a full bladder for them to get a good view and that has always been a struggle for me (holding my bladder that is) since a hysterectomy in 1997 for endometriosis.

After the ultrasound, I was advised that there was a mass on my left ovary which was probably the burst ovarian cyst and buildup of blood and not to worry. However, I was referred to a gynaecologist for an internal ultrasound (oh joy!) and further investigation. She confirmed that there was a mass on my left ovary and that she couldn't rule out ovarian cancer. 'Ovarian cancer says I', 'aren't we rather overacting here?' They do that a bit in Hong Kong I find, even if you have a heavy cold you do sometimes end up in hospital, so was a bit skeptical. How wrong was I, but that was to come later.

I also allowed her to do a CA 125 protein blood test to see if my level was high. This is the marker to measure ovarian cancer. This is not always reliable though as some ovarian cancers express the CA 125 protein and some don't. So, some ladies with a raised level may not have ovarian cancer and vice versa. Mine should have been over 35 but it read as 24.

The doctor however was still a bit twitchy. Anyway, I refused to go further with any more tests as I felt fine. Then I happened to be talking to a colleague at work who said 'I know a very good gynaecological oncology surgeon who is very non-invasive and he'll only operate if he really must'.

I thought 'OK why not I'll go along and see him'. This happened to be on my birthday as we used to get a day's holiday for birthday leave, and my mum accompanied me. He did an internal ultrasound too and said, 'Hmm, I don't like the look of it, if I were you, I'd have it out. We can probably do keyhole surgery. If there's not too much scarring from your previous hysterectomy you'll be up and out in about 4 days'.

I am absolutely blessed to have brilliant medical insurance cover through my job and I know without that I may not still be alive today (but we will come on to that later). We then went through the motions of did I want a general ward, semi private room or private room and that he would open me up and send the tumour down to the lab for analysis and wait half an hour for the result. If all was OK I'd be out of theatre quite quickly, but if he found cancer then he would do what is called full de-bulking, when he would remove all surrounding lymph nodes and all my ovaries, fallopian tubes etc. Therefore if the surgery was keyhole it would only take a few hours.

With all that organised I was booked in for surgery fairly quickly on 6th April 2014 at The Canossa Hospital in a semi private room. With the private medical insurance in Hong Kong you can apply to get a Guarantee of Payment, whereby you get your surgeon/the hospital to confirm all their charges for the treatment. Send these to the insurer who then sends a Guarantee of Payment letter to the hospital to confirm that they will honour payment for the treatment up to the amount you have supplied to them. That way you don't need to pay first and claim back, particularly if you are being admitted for very expensive surgery or treatment.

Down I went for surgery at around 8am on the Monday morning and when I came round looked at the clock and saw that it was early afternoon. 'Hmm, I thought, that doesn't look good'. I also realised that I'd had keyhole surgery so everything should have been very quick.

When my surgeon came to see me he looked very grim and said 'I'm sorry it's ovarian cancer. It's endometrioid cancer with a clear cell component. Because it is clear cell which is very rare and very aggressive, we need to give you chemotherapy treatment. I've cured patients with stage 1 or even stage 2 cancer so let's see what the results are from the other tissue before we discuss the next steps'. As I was recovering from the surgery I just shrugged it off. To be honest, I'm not one for tears and hysteria. 'Oh, my god, I've got cancer' and all that. In fact, nowadays I tend to get tearful at good news since it's so rare to have this!

When he got the results 2 days later he came in on that ward visit with a big smile on his face and said 'Phew, it hasn't spread! You are stage 1, Figo grade 2. The chemotherapy will be what we call adjuvant chemotherapy, which is basically to target any microscopic cells that we can't see to ensure that it doesn't come back. You will need 6 cycles, but I will get an oncologist I know to come and see you in hospital to discuss it all'.

I insisted that my brother be here for that visit and had tried to shield my then 85 year old mother, who had just emigrated out to Hong Kong to be close to family, from the news. As it is, I'm very glad she is here with me as she keeps me going and keeps me strong and the poem at the front of this book is dedicated to her.

A lovely oncologist came to see me and my brother; I have learnt that is always best to have someone with you for these types of conversations as you yourself are so concerned with asking questions, thinking ahead, that you don't always take things in. If you can record the conversation this is always good. In fact, that's what I tell my fellow cancer thrivers, and we still always do on our phones every time we have a consultation with a new doctor that discusses treatment/test results, as it's so useful to play back as a reminder.

This particular oncologist had done time at the Royal Marsden Hospital in London, one of the top cancer hospitals in the world, so I knew I was in good hands.

He explained that I would need 6 cycles of chemotherapy, which would be administered by IV every 3 weeks. This is measured by body weight and as I am quite a big girl being 5 ft. 8" and of 'solid stock', as my mother would say! I needed quite a high dosage. If I knew then what I know now, I would definitely have asked for a lower dosage administered weekly to minimise the side effects, but it's very easy to reflect later!

I was to have 2 drugs, which seem to be standard treatment for ovarian cancer. Paclitaxel, fondly known as Taxol, and Carboplatin. With Paclitaxel, your hair falls out and you can get quite bad peripheral neuropathy (numbness in your fingers and toes). I never suffered from nausea as the drugs they give you are pretty sophisticated these days to keep it at bay, but I suffered from constipation/diarrhoea on and off.

The oncologist advised that one of the major side effects would be incredible fatigue, and that as the drugs built up in my system I may become so ill and immobile that I would be unable to work. This came as a big blow as I love my job and wished to continue working.

When it was time for me to be discharged from the hospital, which happened to be on a Saturday, the accounts department called down to the nurses and advised that my Guarantee of Payment may not be enough to cover the treatment and I may have an outstanding payment to pay. As you can imagine, I was not happy. I had been admitted since the previous Monday and they had had plenty of time to tell me this was the case, so that I could call my broker to get in touch with the insurance company. But, oh no, they had to wait until a

Saturday, when my broker was on a half day and it would be difficult to get hold of him. It's the last thing you need when you are coming out of hospital after surgery. Anyway due to the fact that I was so angry and upset about it they allowed me to be discharged and said they would claim the money from the insurance in retrospect. When I actually got my bill it wasn't over the GOP amount so I have no idea what they were talking about. I'm afraid this happens a lot so be prepared to do battle with the accounts departments in private hospitals if you have private medical care. It's not easy! In Hong Kong, that is the case anyway!

I was busy thinking about work, getting things organised with the medical insurance company and just in general preparing for the chemotherapy treatment, plus recovering from my operation, that I didn't think about whether this disease could kill me, or all the in's and out's as to how rare the clear cell component was, what kind of research was out there into drugs and how to beat this specific aggressive form of ovarian cancer. I didn't really take it all in until much further down my cancer journey. Clear cell ovarian cancer only affects about 6% of women in the western world and here's a piece of interesting information; it affects approximately 25% of women in Japan. No idea why, but they are doing a lot of research into this specific tumour type though. In medical circles, clear cell is known as the long lasting cancer as once you have it, it's difficult to get rid of, which I know only too well! That's where the aggressive term comes from, as in terms of growing fast it's not that active, but you just can't get rid of the darn thing once it gets hold!

One piece of advice, do your research! There is a lot of information on the internet regarding clinical trials etc. (but don't look at the bad stuff out there as everyone is different and don't dwell on the survival rates). From day one I have driven my cancer treatment and will continue to do so! Although I now have an oncologist whose judgement I trust completely. However, I will still challenge if I think I'm unsure about a treatment. As this is your life and your body you are talking about and to be honest oncologists are merely like any doctor, just observers. I do find, though, that here in Hong Kong it is quite rare to find a specialist. Many seem to be all-rounders although there are specialists in breast cancer because more women get this. However many more women die from ovarian cancer.

Anyway I digress! Back to the journey! I then went to see the oncologist in his office and we needed to arrange a Guarantee of Payment with the insurance company to cover my treatment. If you have private insurance, how the doctors deal with the insurance company is hugely important as this is a major factor in treatment. I have put a separate appendix at the back of this book on how to deal with insurance companies as there is specific information and procedures that you need to follow to ensure that everything goes smoothly with your treatment. As mentioned, having that private medical care has probably saved my life so I really can't complain about them. It is tedious dealing with them but the reward is so worth it!

The oncologist, as he was old, just scribbled down costs on a piece of paper and then added more as an afterthought - it was all very ad hoc and just not the right way for me to deal with my insurance company. It had already caused stress and upset and I thought, 'No, don't need this'. So he was dropped quite quickly and my surgeon referred me to another oncologist who wasn't a one-man band and had all the office staff as a back up to assist with paperwork etc. She actually was incredibly arrogant, and also as treatment went on she was quite uncooperative regarding the insurance paperwork as well. I never really trusted her and didn't think she had my welfare at heart, but didn't know anyone else at that time. The oncology clinic, where I am now being treated, was not open at that time so you have to make the best of it sometimes. The aforementioned oncologist 'was fired' by me as well once I had more tumour spread!

Anyway, I was booked in for chemo and off we went. The first treatment was done in the Hong Kong Sanatorium Hospital just in case there might be an allergic reaction and also, I personally prefer the slow drip procedure where you are flushed through with saline after each drug so that the side effects are not so bad. I hadn't realised what else happened to your body when you have chemo i.e. that your white blood cells drop as the chemo kills off good cells as well as malignant cells and this makes your immune system low and open to germs and infections. Also your red blood cells drop and your platelets. So these need to be tested regularly, sometimes weekly, or could be bi-weekly depending on your medical condition and which drugs etc, to ensure that they are OK. If not, you need to inject a white blood cell booster into your leg, in particular, as you are very open to picking up infections, which can be quite dangerous.

For my first session of chemotherapy I didn't really know what to expect, but you basically have a tiny IV tube inserted into a vein in your hand and then depending on the drug (for mine it was 5 to 6 hours) need to wait for the drug or drugs which are mixed with saline, to be infused through into your vein. This shouldn't hurt, but some drugs like my second-round Gemcitabine can burn, but this is normal. For that I just took 2 paracetamol about an hour before treatment so I couldn't feel it.

You are also given oral steroids, anti-histamine drugs and some anti-nausea drugs to ensure that there is no bad reaction to the chemotherapy.

The first day after my treatment I felt OK, just a bit tired, but I did immediately have a nasty rusty metal taste in my mouth (not that I've tasted rusty metal! But it wasn't pleasant!). This was to be expected from the Carboplatin (a platinum based drug) and is a well-known side effect. I drank loads of water and always do after treatment or scans to flush out the toxins, but the water tasted like I was drinking liquid metal, yuck! I read up on this and found that if you add half a lemon juice into the water it really helped which it did funnily enough. I also found that I had a taste for spicy food and all meat tasted ghastly really acidic, so I would make a spicy sauce to go with it and then it tasted OK. The second day I had the most incredible burning in my joints, particularly in my toes, so my dear mum had to massage them and we put a hot water bottle under them to warm them up. After the second day the pain subsided and all was OK. I went back to the office and continued to work so business as usual. Since the chemo was administered every 3 weeks I needed to go back in-between the treatment to get my blood levels tested. As mentioned, I hadn't realised how much time this cancer lark takes up. I sometimes write this book as I wait to see doctors for various tests or results as this can be hours that you are waiting around. Another bit of advice, be prepared for this. Be prepared to spend a lot of time visiting doctors and going for tests and these increase the longer you are taking more drugs, as there is no doubt that although the drugs kill the cancer they also damage the body.

So my routine was set. Every 3 weeks chemo and I realised that the side effects kicked in after a couple of days, so routine was chemo on a Friday afternoon and I then took Monday as sick leave, as this was the worst day for side effects. Going forward the drugs did build up in the body, so the sick days became more frequent and for a longer period, but again that's something that we all have to accept.

About 6 weeks after the treatment started I was warned that I would lose my hair, but I hadn't realised it just suddenly goes! When it was at around that time I thought to myself that I'd better carry a scarf in my bag just in case it starts to fall out. I thought it would just start slowly, but no it was like a big moult! I was sitting on the ferry going to work with my friend when we noticed a bit of hair on my shoulders which I brushed off. But when I got to work and went straight in to a meeting, as I left, the floor was just covered in my hair! I then went to brush it in the ladies' washroom and it just came out in handfuls! I truly hadn't realised it would fall out like this! I immediately booked an appointment with my hairdresser that evening to have it all shaved off. My surgeon had advised this, that once it goes it can be quite distressing, pulling your hair out in handfuls. Distressing my foot! Just the practicality of trying to eat your lunch or have a cup of tea and finding bits of hair everywhere was very inconvenient!

I'm just not a wig person so went the chemo hat, turban or scarf route. Although I did find it quite difficult with the hot weather, as a sensitive bald head can get quite sun burnt just under a thin scarf! So I did need to watch out for the sun!

I also didn't realise that I would lose my eyebrows and eyelashes. In hot weather, it's a bit tricky losing your eyebrows as they perform a very useful function, in the fact that they stop the sweat dripping down from your forehead into your eyes, so again this was an interesting development! The joy of not having to shave legs, underarms or pubes were a definite benefit and saving money by not going to the hairdressers too! I know some women think having a bald head defeminises you, but I never felt that way, I thought it was quite funky.......

I also suffered from very strange and horrible hallucinations. Our helper or mum might be going towards the kitchen and I would visualise them using the blender and cutting off their fingers or lighting the gas on the hob and catching their sleeve and going up in flames. This also continued into dreams, when I would have horrible nightmares when nasty accidents would happen to my mum or brother. Very unpleasant and I assume drug induced. It is the first time that I have actually spoken (or written about this) but it was horrible. This only happened while I was on the chemotherapy, so thankfully I don't have anything like that now.

We continued with the treatments. My bloods went up and down as expected. When the white bloods dropped, I injected a white blood cell booster to bump them back up. Straightforward if you are not squeamish, as mentioned before, it just gets injected into the leg. When the white bloods drop, you do need to be wary of germs and so wearing a face mask is a good idea, or avoiding anyone who is sick. I used to check the health of people coming to meetings so that if anyone had a bad cold or something then I would dial in via Skype for the meeting rather than be in the same room as them. If the platelets drop my oncologist had a good tip and that was to use peanut skins, which funnily enough have great properties for increasing platelet count. It may seem a bit of an odd thing to use, but it does really work. I still use them now with my current treatment. A couple of handfuls fully washed in a cup of boiling water, leave them to steep and then drain them off, and then add half a lemon and a bit of organic honey. We also boil up peanut water and then use it to boil potatoes in it and rice, and adding it in to soups – it all helps with keeping the platelets up. I'll come on to why I do it, but as I inject Clexane (or heparin) a blood thinner, daily into my leg, my platelets cannot fall below 50 so it is important that I keep the levels up for these.

I think the one thing that I really struggled with was the peripheral neuropathy. Our family on my father's side do tend to have strokes and my dear father had a disease called cerebella ataxia which attacks your nervous system – so I think perhaps we are more susceptible to nerve damage. Anyway, the numbness got to a point where my grip went and it was difficult typing on my computer. In my legs it went up as far as my knees, so that I could hardly walk and shuffled along with a walking stick. It's very hard when you can't feel your toes, especially trying to navigate steps as you can't feel the edge very well! Swimming is great to get some exercise as you aren't constantly off balance then.

After cycle four of the chemo my red bloods dropped low and my oncologist gave me a red blood cell booster. For every drug I've received, I've asked for the literature so that I can read up on details of what the side effects are. For this drug, it specifically said beware of blood clotting and DVT. I mentioned this to my oncologist but she pooh poohed my comments. Chemo and specifically clear cell tumours do cause blood clotting also, so however tired you feel it is crucial that you try to exercise and at least move your legs somehow. That's why swimming is so good.

Anyway, the week after the red blood booster I had quite a lot of pain in my lower back and down my left leg. I have in the past suffered from sciatica so thought 'Oh dear, I've got that again' and so just tried to exercise and ease it out. Then my leg seemed to feel really stiff and rigid at the back like the muscles were constantly in cramp and then it eventually became really swollen. This happened over a couple of days. Not being one to make a fuss and worry at every little problem I hadn't really done anything about it, but then decided that perhaps I'd better pop in and see my oncologist. She took one look at my leg and said, 'Oh dear, I think you have a DVT, you need to go and get an ultrasound done immediately this is really urgent'. I looked at her and said 'I told you the injection last week said it might cause blood clots'? To which I got silence! So off I went to hospital; the Canossa again to have an ultrasound. The clot was above my left knee and this meant that I needed to be admitted to hospital, put straight on an IV of heparin and then, I didn't realise but needed to stay in the hospital for 7 days! After consulting with my brother this is standard as he's had a PE (pulmonary embolism) also. But at the time I was on the phone to my oncologist, '7 DAYS, 7 DAYS! You must be joking I have a really important project I need to deliver'. But this is a fact of life with cancer. You have all these unexpected things that happen and then you end being admitted into hospital for treatment. How anyone can say 'Don't let cancer take over or own you' they have to be living in a bubble, because no matter how hard you try, it does! Just from the sheer time spent on medical treatment without even thinking about the mental side of things.

Because my backache was so severe and went down my left leg my oncologist wanted to give me an MRI scan as well just to double check. I am very claustrophobic and when they tried first time it was so small it was like being in an enclosed coffin. Horrible! The nurses gave me a relaxant so that I could be dopey and even drift off to sleep to have it done. Unfortunately they didn't give this enough time to kick in so when I was wheeled down again to try I still couldn't do it. After that I refused. I then, of course, went right off to sleep once back in my room, as the relaxant took it's effect! All the pain was in fact due to the DVT as once the heparin took effect the pain went completely, so I don't think it was anything to do with my back at that time.

I was in a semi private room once again this time and sharing with a lovely Japanese lady who has since become a wonderful friend. We found out that she owned a house in Discovery Bay and had so much to talk about. This cancer journey is hard, but I have to say that I have made so many wonderful friends along the way (I've also sadly lost some too who couldn't handle it), that this has been the one big positive with having this disease.

She had a problem with her back so we had such a laugh; me hobbling around with a stick and she hobbling around with her bad back! My leg did actually become very painful, but as the heparin kicked in became less so and the swelling went down. I had the lovely compression stockings that you are given to keep the circulation going round so looked hilarious. No hair, with these wonderful (I don't think so) white stockings, hobbling around with a stick!

The Canossa Hospital has nuns living in as it is a religious hospital and gets a lot of funding from charitable donations. I remember one of the sisters, Sister Mary, she had breast cancer and was also having dialysis, but she was lovely and had visited me after my surgery last time. She actually remembered me, which was so nice and we had so many good chats each day she visited. I'm not a religious person, although I think I am probably much more in touch spiritually with God now than I've ever been, as I do have a lot to thank him for, it was very nice to have them there and have the daily visits. Her comment was that I was always so bright and positive. I always try to stay that way and to me, as I mentioned before, have found this damn cancer an inconvenience rather than an illness. Although, as it's progressed as time has gone on, I have come to accept that I am really ill (although I've never had any pain from the tumours) and this disease will eventually kill me, unless there is some miracle cure that comes along soon.

While I was in hospital I also had a blood transfusion, and my albumin (protein) topped up. This is usual as these are part of the bloods that drop and get messed up by the chemo.

We were able to drop my heparin down to off the IV, with twice daily injections into my stomach, which was great as I had more freedom to walk around.

My brother and I also had a conversation regarding treatment going forward and it was decided that we would drop the Taxol, so just have the 4 cycles of this drug and carry on with the Carboplatin. The Taxol was just killing my body, and also the peripheral neuropathy after the DVT was just not manageable.

You don't have a crystal ball, but I would have done things oh so differently, had I known then what I know now! But that's why I hope this book will help with imparting information.

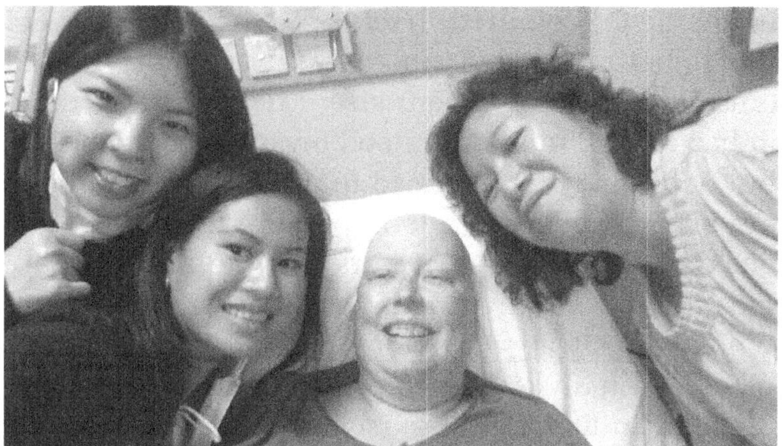

My team who came to visit me in hospital for the first DVT

I was told that I needed to wear the compression stockings all the time which was a nightmare. For small people they have like a kind of belt that goes round your waist and you can clip them to it to hold them up, but for me, forget it! I was far too tall and rotund. You do need something strong to hold them up as they are, after all, compression stockings. I cut the top off mine to get rid of the press stud bit, but then the tops would fall down and flap around and look very odd. I had to purchase lots of long flowing dresses and skirts so you couldn't see the stockings or the top bits flopping around. I did try to pin the tops to my knickers, but because they are so strong they ripped out of my knickers so I am to this day left with lots of pairs of knickers with holes torn in them at the side. These are worn when I am bumming around the house in my casual clothes, as it seems a waste to just throw them away! In the end I found a company in UK who made flesh coloured hold up type, which were much better, stayed up themselves, didn't stand out and were in a decent size. I used to wear them in bed as had misunderstood my oncologist on this, but actually you only need to wear them when you are sitting down for a long period of time i.e. At a desk or flying, since if you are walking you are moving around, or in bed your legs are raised up. When I am sitting down for a period of time, in most places I will always try to put my feet up. Now I am on heparin lifelong there is very little chance of me having a blood clot, so I no longer wear the stockings. Only for flying which is a different situation totally.

We continued with the 2 final cycles of the Carboplatin and that was that. When I saw my oncologist for a final follow up appointment and asked what follow up I should have, her response was 'Well, you never really had it my dear'. I know the chemotherapy was adjuvant, but still no advice on diet, no advice on supplements, nothing! I am MUCH wiser and more informed now. As I say, you can't turn back the clock but had I been more informed at the start of my treatment I would have done things very differently! I know I keep saying this and that's why I hope this book will help other patients with cancer, to impart knowledge, to give you the opportunity to make better and informed decisions earlier in your journey.

So that was that! I continued with the supplements that I would take anyway, like Vitamin C and the B12 for the nerve damage at the end of my fingers and toes and continued with life. My hair grew back gradually and was just so soft! Soft as a baby's! and really curly! This is fondly known as the chemo curl and happens when you have your head shaved or your hair falls out, apparently!

While having treatment at the clinic I met a wonderful Chinese lady called Crane (like the bird). She had stage 4 colon cancer that had metastasised into her liver. She was so bubbly and positive that we eventually exchanged phone numbers and became good friends. She was an investment banker, single mum, separated from her husband, with her grown up son living in the UK, and sisters in the States and parents in China. I always thought she didn't have such a strong support system which is so important. After a bad scan result she said she often felt lonely, which is awful. No one should ever have to go through this alone EVER. I am very blessed that my mum lives with me and I have my brother and sister in law close by, plus so many great and close friends.

Crane introduced me to a lot of alternative treatments that I took with a fair amount of skepticism. Drinking tea made from the leaves of the Soursop tree didn't really do it for me, or using purified water and tapping (EFT) to minimise stress. But my mind set has really been changed on this, which I will come on to later. We used to sit together when having our chemo and I can clearly remember her saying 'I can't believe I might die' with her eyes welling up with tears. Crane spent a traditional English Christmas with us that December in 2014, but passed away in a clinic in Germany the following Easter Monday. I still miss her terribly, as we would have had so much to share and talk about. I have never really cried about having my cancer, but the day I heard about Crane I did cry, for her and what a waste of a beautiful life with so much to live for. A few other of my fellow cancer warriors have since passed away and to me that's the hardest thing. It is inevitable in some cases. But we all so want to live! For our families, for our friends, for our kids, for our grandkids. It makes you see how precious life is; enjoy every day for you truly don't know how long you have got!

So life continued. My bloods were checked every 3 weeks and I was booked in for a PET scan the following February (2015).

February came and off I went for my PET scan, or Positive Emission Tomography to give it, its proper name. These have now become routine (I'm sad to say), but you have to be a bit careful as to how often you have them due to the radioactivity, and also I feel sometimes you can go looking for things! The PET scan is an interesting experience and something that you need to plan at least a half day for.

You have to fast for 6 hours before hand, so it's good if you can get an early appointment, like 9am. You are once again given an IV line in your hand and also your glucose level is usually tested. A radioactive dye together with glucose is injected through the line. You then have to wait for about an hour; you are left in a private room due to the radioactivity, with a comfortable bed or reclining chair to rest in and then called in to the scan about an hour later. When I had them done in the Hong Kong Sanatorium the radiologist always wanted me to insert a tampon as I have no womb, so that he could track where everything was. The first PET scan the nurse was asking lots of different questions and I didn't catch all of them and answered yes to all, as you do! But found myself being offered help to insert the tampon! 'Oooh no, that's fine I said, just let me know when you want me to do it and I'll pop it in, not a problem'! I have since been through some humiliating medical things, but inserting a tampon was definitely something I can do on my own. Thank you very much! Although I have to say once you go through menopause you do get a bit dry in your nether regions so it's not that pleasant without a bit of lubrication. Probably a bit too much information there! But we cancer thrivers do find that we talk about our stomach and other areas down below a lot, particularly our bowels!!

After the hour, I was asked to drink a cup of water and was then called in. I don't mind the PET scan at all as it's like a large donut. Nothing like an MRI scan when you feel you are in a horrible enclosed coffin and it's so noisy! The PET scan is much more civilised!

After the scan is finished you need to wait until they check it is OK, and then you need to wait an hour or so for the radioactivity to become safe. You are then told not to go near young babies or pregnant women for 8 hours or so.

The tumour activity is measured by its SUV (standardised uptake value) and this can vary per organ. For instance, the SUV threshold in the lungs is lower than in the liver. For my scan, it's the SUV normal uptake in the liver which is measured, so this can vary. Please refer to my PET scan results in the appendix. If you look at your scan you can see that the active tumours are usually glowing very brightly as they have taken up the radioactive glucose quickly. However, sometimes this can also be inflammation instead, so your oncologist and radiologist need to look at your medical history. If you have active cancer then it is more than likely to be active cancer. But the back vertebra bone marrow can glow and the brain and other areas of the body that are not malignant, so it does take an expert to interpret the scans properly.

Then came the horrible wait that all us cancer thrivers call scanxiety, which for me has increased as my cancer has slowly spread. The radiologist gives nothing away and you need to wait until the oncologist receives the report to get the results. In Hong Kong with the luxury of private medical insurance you can get this within 2 days, which is really good.

Off I went to see the oncologist and she said there was a very small peritoneal nodule that had appeared, so basically a small nodule in my abdomen. But it wasn't malignant and so she decided to do a 'watch and wait' strategy. I also saw my surgeon and he said, 'Well, if it does turn malignant you can always have chemotherapy again' so matter of fact about it all! Once again, if I had known then what I know now about clear cell I would have insisted on some kind of treatment to prevent it turning malignant. Perhaps an Aromatase Inhibitor or now I would ask for some kind of immunotherapy vaccine or a targeted drug which weren't available then. More to follow later on this.

Life carried on, I went to the office as usual, had fun with friends and family as usual, my hair had grown back by then and my peripheral neuropathy was much improved so everything was good.

I had regular blood tests, my CA125 marker remained low at 5, I was booked in for another PET scan in May just as a follow up and everything continued.

Chapter Two

The First Recurrence

When May came, off I went to the Hong Kong Sanatorium for the scan and then as always the 2 day wait for the results.

My surgeon also got copies of the scan and I remember the day after that getting a call from his clinic. I was in a meeting in the office, which I stepped out of, and his receptionist said 'You need to see your oncologist, the cancer is back, you have 2 tumours in your abdomen. You need to go back on to chemotherapy'. I'm afraid I did burst into tears at that point and hugged my dear friend Anne-Marie, as the thought then of going back on chemo seemed daunting, and as I hadn't actually seen the scan I didn't really know what we were dealing with.

When I saw the oncologist she explained that the original tumour had turned malignant, and I also had one in an iliac node near my hip. They were small and there was no spread anywhere else so that at least was a blessing. I didn't like the fact that the peritoneal nodule was quite close to my liver, as my one big concern was that the cancer would spread into major organs, and then we would be in trouble. But it was what it was.

I had also at this time been suffering from excruciating back ache, which after an x-ray my GP thought was a prolapsed disc, and I visited a wonderful chiropractor called Dr Michael Back! Loved the name and he was really good! But later we actually found that the iliac tumour was pressing on a nerve and causing the pain, which was interesting! Once it was removed the pain disappeared immediately. He did give me some fantastic treatment, but it didn't last long obviously because of the tumour.

We had discussions, my surgeon and my oncologist and I. As mentioned previously I had begun to mistrust my oncologist, just because she was so incredibly arrogant and wouldn't listen to me. If I asked a perfectly normal question she would just shrug her shoulders and look down her nose. I complained to my surgeon about her, but he said she has cured some very sick cancer patients, so at the time I was so tired that I decided to stick with her. A word of advice when you start this journey, choose an oncologist that you trust completely, and one that you know has your wellbeing and interest at heart. A lot of oncologists I have found don't, and for sure out here, as everything runs on private medical insurance, many are driven by money! If I had my time over I would also choose a younger oncologist, as they are more up on the latest drugs and treatments. Also ones that are recommended from other cancer patients under their care are normally a safe bet.

So my oncologist recommended 2nd line chemotherapy, which is when the next line of suggested drugs for your kind of cancer come into play. A lot of oncologists here in Hong Kong, as previously mentioned, are not experts in ovarian cancer but more all-rounders. If they are specialists in women's cancer it is usually breast cancer. So I sought advice from a consultant medical oncologist in Bath my home town in the UK. She was a specialist in ovarian cancer so I could bounce ideas off her and gain reassurance that this would be the route that she would go down too. I also consulted with my surgeon, once again taking my brother with me to digest any information, as I would miss half the conversation being too emotionally involved! Out here they never discuss about the future and when I raised this my surgeon said 'Don't think about it otherwise you will be in a very dark place! The good thing is the cancer is contained in your abdomen and because the tumours are so small you have time on your side'.

We started the new treatment with 2 drugs: Capecitabine (brand name Xeloda) was taken orally in the form of 10 tablets a day, and Gemcitabine administered by IV every 3 weeks.

I think I mentioned that for my first treatment of Gemcitabine I had a horrible burning through my veins which I was told was normal, and was given Panadol. A bit too late the first time! But after that I came prepared and had already taken it beforehand. The Capecitabine gave me awful, awful diarrhoea and after the first week of taking it gave me bleeding gums, which was rather unpleasant. However, our next door neighbour back home in

Bath, who was an oncology pharmacist, advised that a great mouthwash called Difflam Forte was good for helping with sore and bleeding gums. I used this and also brushed my teeth with a soft children's toothbrush, plus upped my vitamin C intake, and this did disappear after a couple of weeks and I've never had bleeding gums again after that episode. She also thought that taking 10 tablets a day of Capecitabine was too much. I know the dose is calculated on body weight and I'm a big girl, but due to the diarrhoea she said it seemed too much. My oncologist agreed to drop the dose to 8 tablets a day which seemed better.

Life carried on and my oncologist said she would scan after 2 cycles. At this time I got a phone call from a wonderful lady who ran a cancer support group for English speaking women in Hong Kong (there are many groups for local Cantonese speaking) who said she was friends with Crane and had heard about me from her. Crane had at that time just recently died, so we were able to share information about that also. Her sister arranged a memorial for her, which we never got to attend as we never knew about it, and I will always regret that I never got the chance to say goodbye properly, but she will always remain in my heart for as long as I am still alive, so I suppose that's what counts. The support group is called Cancer Connect and I have shared details in the appendix, but this group was a godsend for me. Full of ladies who had, or were going through, cancer treatment, knew how tough chemo was and all the trials and tribulations of having cancer. I can advise anyone with cancer to find a support group as you will never feel lonely and will always have that support to get you through the bad days. There are also some good internet support groups out there, full of information (sometimes too much), so it's always useful to join some of them. However the face to face contact, especially having visits in hospital, are so important.

Cancer Connect meets the first Wednesday of every month for a coffee morning and there is always a Christmas get together, which is nice. Ladies tend to break out and those with the same interests tend to bond together. I have some very good friends from that group who I know will be friends for life.

I also at that time met a lady in the taxi queue one day who worked in the same office complex on Hong Kong island as me and we shared a taxi. She now must be one of my dearest and closest friends here; my cancer has definitely brought us together and I am so grateful for her amazing friendship and support. So this disease is not all bad, I have truly made some amazing friendships through having this disease for sure. Sara also has a wonderful Dalmatian called Ella, who I absolutely adore and when I was having a bad time I only had to give Ella a cuddle and she would make me feel so much better. Animals are such a great therapy when you are feeling down or ill. They seem to sense your pain and just want to give unconditional love.

Although Ella, like all dogs, is rather driven by her stomach and she does know that Auntie Hilary will bring her a treat or two!

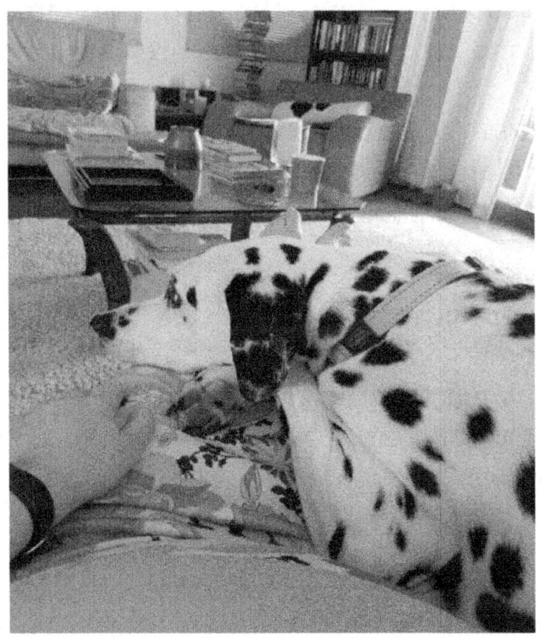

Dear lovely Ella sitting on my lap

After 2 cycles, as promised, off I went for a PET scan to see if the chemo mix was working. The scan came back as clear, and we were all very excited that this combination was working and we were finally going to knock it on the head. It is always a boost when you see that all the discomfort is worth it! So we continued with four more cycles of the Gem Cap therapy.

Unfortunately, a few weeks into the third cycle I could see that my right leg was a bit swollen again and thought 'Oh no, I'd better go and get it checked out earlier this time!' My oncologist was on a cruise and uncontactable and so I saw another doctor in her practice. He took a look and said 'Sorry it looks like another DVT. You'd better go and have an ultrasound done'. Yes, it was conclusive; another DVT, so off I was rushed to the Canossa Hospital again! As luck would have it, since my oncologist was away I saw another blood oncologist, a specialist in anything blood related, whether cancer or blood clots, and he is fantastic. All the nurses kept saying, 'Oh, he's very serious all the time but when you see him on the phone to his daughter he is like a teddy bear, laughing and joking'. It became my mission to make him laugh every day when he came to see me and I did! The nurses thought this was amazing! When I was admitted I also developed a cough which he didn't like the sound of and I had to have a CT to check this. We found that I also had a few blood clots in my lungs which was a pulmonary embolism! But, same treatment, 7 days in hospital; he did everything by injection in the tummy rather than an IV drip which was much easier as I could move around more freely.

I remember when I arrived I was put into a semi private room again, this time with an old lady. I thought 'That looks OK she'll be very quiet'. But when she came around from the anaesthetic, my god, all she did was yell at intervals! I didn't get any sleep the first night and said to the nurses 'Sorry get me out of here and into another room. I won't survive a week of this! She needs to be in a private room!!!' I got moved next door which was much better, although the bathrooms are backing onto each other, so when I was having a shower or using the loo I could still hear her yelling away! All good fun! They did apologise and say 'Sorry we didn't realise she would be that noisy' but were, as always, quick to charge me 50 pounds for a change of room!

The wonderful sister came on her rounds and said 'Hello again!' And we had a good chat. I do often wonder if she is still there and she is still as well as she can be. My last surgery was done in a different hospital as my surgeon operated there rather than the Canossa Hospital. They all have their favourite hospitals!

Once I got discharged from the Canossa I was then to inject heparin for life into my leg, as two DVT's and a pulmonary embolism was too much of a risk to leave it.

After my first DVT my surgeon did question why I wasn't put on blood thinners then, but my oncologist said that if I started taking them then I would be on them for life. Should have listened to my surgeon!

I do know some oncologists will put clear cell cancer patients on blood thinners right away, as the risk of having a DVT is very high with clear cell tumours. My brother takes tablets after having his

PE, but my wonderful blood oncologist says that injecting is far more effective. He also says that there is a very low risk that I will ever get another DVT/PE now I'm on heparin, which is re-assuring. I just have to monitor my platelets and make sure they stay above 50 otherwise I will get bleeding.

During the Gem Cap treatment, I put on loads of weight and got what they call a 'moon face' when your face swells up and becomes very round. I hadn't realised how bad it had got until I saw a photo of myself. It was uncomfortable actually as it's not nice having your skin stretch on your face. I also had visions of loads of wrinkles, as the swelling went down in due course when I came off the drugs and lost about 27 lbs in 2 weeks! That didn't happen, thankfully! I did get the inevitable stretch marks on my tummy and thighs though, but after having a lot of surgery since, there is no way these parts of the body will be exposed to anyone publicly nowadays!

I also developed a bit of what's called hand and foot syndrome, which is when you get very cracked and dry hands and feet, caused particularly by the Gem Cap therapy. The oncologist in Bath recommended a wonderful cream called Udderly Smooth with UREA, that was designed to put on cow's sore udders and worked a treat. It didn't cost much and was available on Amazon.

At this time I was very positive mentally, but found that I would be in tears over small things. An urgent e-mail wouldn't send for work as the wi-fi at home started playing up, or I banged my head on a kitchen cupboard one time and went running off in tears. I guess in retrospect these were also reflective of my feelings on the bigger picture, but just came out differently. This journey is such a rollercoaster mentally and physically that you have to be strong to survive it and make the best of it that you can. Yes! Absolutely there are dark days, usually when the side effects are unmanageable or after bad scan results, but you have to accept that it is what it is and tomorrow is another day. If you don't, trust me, it will destroy you......

One of the most embarrassing side effects and apparently very usual with this drug combination, was uncontrollable wind which was also quite, let's say, fragrant to say the least!

When I went to take the ferry over to Hong Kong for my checkups I would think dogs and babies; sit by dogs and babies and then when a small fart quietly slipped out I could look disapprovingly at them holding my head up high, ME, no that wasn't me!

On one occasion, which was so funny, but probably won't seem that way as I write it, I was coming home in rush hour after a late oncologist's appointment. Everyone on the ferry always runs for the front gangway seats next to the doors, so they can rush off at the other end. These seats as they are front gangway seats, are also best for people like me at that time walking with a stick, as they are close to the door and with more leg room. Anyway, on this occasion I was sitting on a very busy ferry in the front row seats and, I'm afraid, a rather windy day in the bowel department for some reason. Some very smelly farts slipped out, nothing I can do about it, but I've never seen that front row clear so fast of people! It was embarrassing at the time, but now I have to chuckle! You've just got to laugh at these things as they become a way of life after a while. If you didn't see the funny side you would really be destroyed by what this disease throws at you, as I said before.

At this time and belatedly, I know, I realised that diet and supplements had a big part to play in keeping well and even some clinical studies have shown that some herbs, vegetables and spices can really promote apoptosis (cancer cell death).

I haven't eaten wheat for many years as my father was a coeliac, and I've always had an intolerance to wheat. A GI-MAP stool test also confirmed my gluten intolerance. I also used to suffer from really bad catarrh and sinus problems so didn't have any dairy and drank soya milk and ate goats cheese. I also, because of migraines, didn't drink caffeine or much alcohol. I was very much a lover of raw salads, steamed fish and chicken and not a huge red meat eater, although I do like a good steak – this is now organic, grass fed, antibiotic and added hormone free. I was a lover of crisps in any shape or form, not a lover of cakes and biscuits or chocolate, except the dark kind, but I did love my crisps.

After reading up on diet I saw that gluten, dairy, soya milk could cause inflammation in the body and, of course, things like processed foods, where all the goodness is processed out, or canned goods that have added salt were not good. Certain cooking oils can give off toxic carcinogens when heated to certain levels, so I switched to coconut oil or olive oil or ghee as they seemed to be the best. All processed sugary items were off the menu, I think it is widely known that sugar contains glucose which cancer feeds on. This is very evident when you have a PET scan, which uses radioactive glucose, which the tumours immediately absorb and then glow on the scan. Although inflammation can also glow on a scan, not only malignant tumours. However, there is as yet no detailed clinical research to prove that sugar can encourage cancer to grow, as good cells also need glucose to repair and grow, so my rule of thumb was to eat fruit and good carbs and then just cut out all the processed stuff. I also stopped soya milk as this seems to cause inflammation and switched to coconut milk. Then I read up on hemp milk, which seemed even more healthy. It took me a while to find the right one, but I now wouldn't be without it. It gives me a chuckle that my ideal hemp milk comes from a little farm in Devon, UK! All the way to Hong Kong.

All fried food and microwaving was out. Processed salt or sugar were replaced with Himalayan pink salt and raw coconut sugar, all vegetables became organic and fruit where possible, white rice became white Basmati rice as less processed, or brown or red rice. I would make raw juice to get lots of goodness from this, all meat was organic and as I mentioned previously, added hormone free, antibiotic free, free range.

I guess everyone ends up having their favourite cookbooks, so some of mine are listed in the appendix but I found The Nourish Cookbook by the Penny Brohn Foundation very useful for a beginner. She came to talk to my mum's Graduate Women's group many years ago when in remission, as she had breast cancer, and mum remarked on how lively and funny she was. Unfortunately, she did pass away in the end, but had set up the Penny Brohn Centre, which is close to my home town in Bath. It is a place of tranquility to go to for advice and support for cancer patients. I find you have to get into your own routine on your food though. There are so many anti -cancer diets out there so you need to decide what works for you. 'I cured myself of stage 4 cancer by eating raw food and juicing vegetables' just doesn't do it for me, I'm afraid, and if you are deluded enough to believe that then that's your decision! With an aggressive cancer like clear cell, yes diet helps you to feel well and keep your body strong, but cure this type of cancer, nah!

I also looked into taking more supplements, but you really, really have to be careful with this, as I have found out to my cost (both financially and with drug interactions). You really need to know what you are doing, otherwise you can get some herbs and supplements that interfere with drug efficacy. We are going through some horrible side effects anyway, the last thing you want to do is to stop the drugs working by interfering with their effectiveness through using supplements. If you have an iPhone there is a great app from Sloane Kettering Cancer Hospital in USA called 'About Herbs' and it lists all the supplements and herbs and what they can do for cancer, plus which cancer drugs and ingredients they interact with. I don't have iPhone only android, but you can just go into their website and get into the link that way. I have put the link in the appendix. I will write later how one supplement I was taking seriously affected my body and seriously affected the absorption of one of my drugs.

Chapter Three

The Second Recurrence

Back to the journey! After 4 more cycles of the Gem Cap treatment we did another PET scan expecting everything to be clear, but no, the 2 tumours had come back with a vengeance, more active and slightly bigger. Since I had no spread anywhere else in the body we discussed at length and it was decided that my surgeon would open me up again, this time across my belly (rather than the previous keyhole) so more painful and more recovery time but at least he could have a good look around inside.

Now a new test had come into play called the Next Generation Sequencing Test by a company called Foundation Medicine in Boston. They basically ask for a tumour sample where they can test the genomic make up of the tumour and then suggest targeted drugs that can be used to combat these mutations. They will look on their data base and list all the clinical trials that are happening for clear cell ovarian cancer, or it may be just for solid tumours, and these can be used as a reference point for treatment. I have listed in the appendix the genomic mutations found in my first test (I have now had 3!), but the most important one to note here is the ARID1A gene, which has been seen to be resistant to platinum based chemotherapy in clear cell cancer patients. So that explains probably (in my mind anyway, I'm not a doctor) why my first line of chemotherapy was not so successful, as I only had 4 cycles of Taxol and the 6 of Carboplatin were ineffective, which means I only really had 4 effective cycles of chemotherapy. You can't look back but there is no way if I was starting this journey now that I would look at chemotherapy as a single agent as my first option! I will come on to how targeted drugs work later.

I decided to treat myself to a private room this time as I knew I was going to have a bit of discomfort when I came out of the surgery. I had to stop my blood thinning drug heparin 3 days before the surgery and had my blood doctor on standby in case of any bleed out.

The one thing I hate about surgery is that your bowel goes to sleep, especially with abdomen surgery, and you can feel it bloating up and the wind moving around which is excruciatingly painful, and until you fart and let it out and the bowel has then started moving you get relief. I have now realised what the trick is for not prolonging this. As soon as you can get up out of bed, have an enema. This gets the bowel moving nicely and gets all the air out. Such a relief. I didn't discover this until my third surgery, but I know now for the future!

Quite a few friends visited and the time and healing passed quite quickly. I did have a nasty experience the day after surgery which has taught me a lesson regarding keeping the call bell close. I had struggled up to use the loo and should have asked a nurse to help me, but really wanted to be independent. I came back and somehow fell awkwardly onto my back on my bed, so half on and half off. Unfortunately, I'd stupidly not put the call bell in reach and couldn't pull myself up. I called out 'Someone help me, help me' and shouted and shouted but no one heard as I was in a private room. I could feel myself slipping off the bed and knew that I had to do something. Because of the angle, I couldn't grab the bed rails properly or raise the back of the bed so the only way to pull myself up was by my stomach muscles. I don't think I have ever screamed so much with pain in my life and was shaking with shock when I righted myself on the bed. Of course, in tears as well. I immediately called the nurses who calmed me down and checked my wound. I will never ever go to the toilet right after surgery without a nurse's assistance in future and will never put the call bell out of reach ever again. Very scary and painful experience. Sometimes you need to accept that you need help and not to try and do it all yourself.

I never saw the lovely nun but I think she only covered the medical wards not the surgical wards, so still don't know how she is faring. Maybe she might read this book and know that I am thinking of her anyway.

For some reason, I developed rather large blisters around where my surgical dressing was on my wound and also on my bottom. Quite funny when you have a group of nurses trying to figure out what to do when you are bending over the sink for them to have a good examine of your backside. Good job the bowel was still waking up otherwise who knows what might have blown out at the wrong moment! In the end, they decided to burst them and use zinc cream to help with the soreness and dry out the skin. It was an allergy to the dressing in the end and also to iodine, as I've had this now several times, so I need a special hypo allergenic dressing whenever I need to have any wounds dressed and to avoid iodine based liquids.

When it came once again to check out, oh yes you've got it, I was checking out on a Sunday and we had the same mess up again with the GOP. This time I had planned ahead and put some extra money on my credit card to cover any more money demands and once again, yes I had an argument with the silly head of accounts for not planning ahead. I was even wheeled up in my wheelchair to go and yell at them. So annoyed. But I dutifully payed the excess on my credit card and was refunded the money, not until a month later, mind you, once the insurance paid the hospital. Nothing to do with my insurance at all, this was all down to the hospital's accounts department. At that point I did say that if I ever needed surgery again there would be no way I was returning to their hospital. And I haven't! it's a shame as the nurses and the nuns were so nice.

My wonderful surgeon told me that he'd got the tumours, they were very small, but he was able to get them. The one in the iliac was buried very deeply and he had to go through what is fondly known as the 'valley of death' between 2 big blood vessels to reach it. He had to keep peeling off layers of lymph nodes to reach it, but was determined to get to it and get it out. I've since been told that many surgeons would not have tried to attempt this, so once again I was very blessed to have such a great surgeon. Also there was no spread once again. My surgeon suggested the next course of action should be adjuvant radiotherapy, just to run it up over the lymph nodes around the abdomen to ensure that we had really got any rogue malignant cells again. Radiotherapy was originally designed for cervical cancers apparently so my surgeon deemed this would be a good route. I also asked him about other patients of his with ovarian cancer and if it had worked for them and he replied 'Yes they were cured'.

My oncologist was up for doing this treatment also but the radiotherapy oncologist I went to see to do it was really reluctant. He said that radiotherapy was quite old fashioned and he suggested more systemic treatment again like chemotherapy, but my answer to his suggestion was that I'd had 2 lines already and each time the cancer had recurred? He then had a case conference with my surgeon and oncologist and then decided to go ahead. I also pushed for it as thought it seemed a good option since the chemotherapy seemed ineffective. I did read a lot of research that advised that having radiotherapy can cause more tumours to grow outside the radiotherapy area at a later date, but was prepared to take the risk. Once again the biggest mistake I have ever made! But you just don't know the right course of action sometimes.

So it was agreed that I would have a month's worth of radiotherapy at the Hong Kong Sanatorium as this has the best equipment. I would need to go in every day.

I have to say this treatment was worse than chemotherapy by far, very grueling and incredibly tiring.

For preparation they needed to measure a few things, which was a very interesting experience! If anyone had been a fly on the wall that day I think they would have had a few chuckles!

For radiotherapy for ovarian cancer the oncologist needs you to have a full bladder, which then pushes the bowel out the way to minimise radiation to this. It can get very inflamed and also get fibrosis (thickening of the bowel wall) which can cause a blockage if it is exposed to too much radiation, so it is important to protect it.

In order to measure how much liquid needs to be in the bladder this needs to be done by filling the bladder with saline.

I remember this afternoon well! Me lying on the CT scanner bed. A tube going into the bladder and then it being filled with saline, my oncologist saying, 'The nurse has heated it first so it will be nice and warm', a tube up my bottom to measure from that side. My oncologist stood with a metal container letting the coloured dye run inside my bowel, quite happily having a jolly conversation with me. Mamas and Papas singing 'All the Leaves are Brown' and me singing along and going up an octave when the tubes tickled upon insertion. Once all was filled, me going through the CT scanner with a contrast dye inserted to take measurements. All these lovely young male nurses with very mellow Canadian accents telling me I was doing really well. What a picture it must have been. Then they drew black lines all over my abdomen to do the guides for the radiotherapy machine and covered them with tape so they didn't shower off and ready to go.

So basically what I needed to do then before every treatment was drink water an hour before treatment and fill my bladder to a certain level, which was measured when I had the CT prep scan previously which would push the bowel out the way. It was very difficult to measure the level, which was done by ultrasound. Some days I would feel like my bladder was going to burst and other days it didn't feel too bad. But once the bladder was full I would then have to go under the radiotherapy machine for 30 minutes and not move. If I was desperate for a wee before I started the treatment you can imagine how I felt at the end. I would be running out of the room with my knickers already pulled down! A radiologist holding the toilet door open for me and then relief! Sometimes if for some reason there was a delay and when I was measured the nurse would say, 'Oh dear you're really full already, can you hold it for another half hour' to which I would reply, 'You must be joking' and then I would have to empty my bladder and start all over again. I hated that month, everyday having to fill my bladder to the exact measurement, feeling incredibly tired, my white blood cells dropped and I also caught an awful cold with a nasty cough, so was unable to lie still under the machine, making a few treatments delayed.

I also went for regular checks with my gastroenterologist to ensure that I wasn't going to have any blockages from the radiotherapy. I did get constipation occasionally, for which she told me to always use glycerin suppositories to help, as once the bowel shuts down, even if you eat lots of fruit, take laxatives, these will just give you gas or bloat you up. She was right actually; nothing like a glycerin suppository to get the bowel moving. Likewise, with my bouts of diarrhoea she told me not to use Imodium as that actually stops the bowel from working. Then you get constipated the day after, while with another drug called Duspatalin this just stops the bowel from cramping, slows it down and stops it that way. Again she was correct and that's what I use for bouts of diarrhoea.

Chapter Four

The Third Recurrence

Once the radiotherapy was completed we let it settle for a few weeks and then I went for a PET scan. Nothing to worry about really, except the radiographer came out and said 'I'll just put this strap across your chest to hold in your breasts', which was odd as I've never had that done before (after the news received later, I can see now that she wanted a better view of my liver!).

So, all done and dusted and then that horrible wait for the results. I went on my own, as I thought this is only a follow up and the radiotherapy will have done the trick and we are now all clear BUT how wrong was I!!! Never second guess this damn clear cell cancer as it's always one step ahead of you!

I walked into the oncologist's room and there hanging up on the lightbox was my scan result. I could see a massive tumour in the liver and also what looked like 6 other smaller ones. All my oncologist said was 'Yes, you have tumours in your liver and one is really big!' What a reassuring way to speak to a patient (I don't think so!). My only thought was, 'shit, I'm not coming back from this!' When I asked how the spread had happened she retorted, 'It's through the blood of course!' She actually looked really angry and to my mind flustered and didn't know what do. She even phoned the oncologist who'd done the radiotherapy to ask if he'd done a CT scan through my radiotherapy treatment and he said he had but only round the pelvic area. She was laughing and joking with him on the phone and I thought 'HOW DARE YOU'. I'm sitting here in shock and you don't seem to care. So then my questions came, 'What are you going to do? It's clear the chemo isn't working? How about trying a targeted drug, ovarian cancer is highly angiogenic that might work?' To which she replied 'No, you've had a blood clot and are now taking heparin you might have a brain bleed'. 'How about surgery? Can the tumours be removed?' 'No, they are too big'. So I just sat there astounded in shock. 'I want a biopsy done to see what we are dealing with here, by some miracle it may be benign?' 'No, it's obvious it's cancer'. This just went on and then silence again. I just glared at her......then she turned around from her screen and said 'I'm a woman of action me, I'm thinking what we should do next.' Pffffh! That's when I said to myself, 'Nah, you're fired Mrs, you haven't got a clue what to do now!'

Also I must note here that my CA125 marker had remained at 5 since my first line of chemotherapy. Until, a few days before my PET scan when my haematology doctor tested it and it had suddenly jumped up to 140. By then the tumours were of considerable size in my liver, so once again a reminder that some women just can't rely on this marker as a predictor of tumour activity.

Anyway, she agreed that I could have a biopsy done and on the biggest tumour, which was 10cm, you couldn't really miss it! And also I was going to have a porta cath put in. Because we had so many challenges now putting in a line into my veins and because it was clear that I needed to continue with regular treatment this was a way of getting the needle in easily. Basically, a porta cath is a catheter which is inserted under your skin either in your neck with a line going into your carotid artery or in my case just above the left breast and the line goes into an artery near the heart. You then end up with a hard-circular object under your skin and when you have treatment the oncology nurse pushes a needle through the skin and this punctures the catheter and then all drugs are infused through a line going into the catheter. You can also have blood taken through it, but my oncology nurse does say that the catheter has more chance of getting blocked. They take my blood through my arm still. The only thing you need to do is take a deep breath when the needle goes in and take a deep breath when the needle is removed. So much easier than going through all the pain and discomfort of trying to find non- existent veins which have hardened and collapsed due to frequent blood taking and also from chemo treatment. I think the record for finding my veins was 7 attempts, all very painful.

So once again I needed to contact my insurance broker to be admitted to the Hong Kong Sanatorium and a bed was booked.

I went down in the morning and had the biopsy done first. I was so worried, I couldn't think of anything worse than having a needle put into my liver and was so terrified about the pain. However, it wasn't too bad at all. The radiotherapy doctor was great such a soft calming voice!

The procedure basically entails him putting in a local anaesthetic so you don't feel it go through the skin. Then the probe goes in and you feel a bit of a stab in your liver. Then each time he wanted to take a sample I had to breathe in and I felt a very small prick in my liver. He took several samples and then withdrew the probe. He then filled the small hole in the liver with some gel; at this point you feel like you have really painful indigestion, but it literally only lasts about a minute and then done. All this was completed by guided ultrasound, but with the largest tumour being 10cm you couldn't miss it really!

Then in the afternoon I was wheeled down to have my porta cath inserted. This is proper surgery as they need to cut into the skin and insert it underneath, so you usually have a general anaesthetic for this. Although, I know some of my other cancer thrivers have had theirs inserted by their oncologist in the clinic but I prefer the hospital. When I came around it was very sore but otherwise OK.

I was so hungry as I hadn't been allowed to eat for almost all day, so once back on the ward ordered my favourite there, which was steamed garoupa with broccoli.

After about 30 minutes the stomach decided it was all too much! And as they wouldn't let me use the proper toilet (because of the movement) due to risk of liver bleeding, I rushed on to the commode near the bed, and, oh boy, had the biggest poo ever! I was in a general ward as no need for a private room for such small surgery, so I don't know what the other patients thought! It was a struggle for the nurses to even let me have a commode, though as they said 'No, no, no you need to stay still as you've had a biopsy on the liver.' Has anyone ever tried to use a bedpan lying down, if you can you're a better man than me, Gunga Din! I just can't do it as it defies gravity!

Anyway, after that little episode, I only had to wait a couple of hours and was discharged, thank goodness.

I then went back to my wonderful surgeon with my brother for support and showed him my scan, he didn't say much as usual and wasn't about to say 'Oh this is very bad, you have 2 years to live' blah, blah. He was much more upbeat and we discussed if he knew any more oncologists that I could try. If you read statistics for stage 4 clear cell ovarian cancer, which I was now after the spread to the liver, it says that the prognosis is very poor and the survival rate over 5 years is as low as 1-2%, but this is when you have to shut this out and keep going, as everyone is different and I hope that my case is a positive example!! He did say the oncologist I was with currently was well known to be arrogant and not well liked in many circles, 'Well, thanks for telling me that now!' But said as previously mentioned had in fairness cured a lot of sick people.

He didn't discuss surgery either, but said that I needed systemic treatment with some kind of drug as we didn't know really if there were other microscopic cancer cells in other areas of the body. I came off my last round of chemo at the end of the previous year and since the radiotherapy at the beginning of the year hadn't had any drugs to treat the whole body so I could see where he was coming from, I guess. I did also discuss this with the specialist oncologist in the UK and she said that basically the radiotherapy would have lowered my immune system and any microscopic cells outside the radiation area would have been 'Having a party!' as I'd had no systemic treatment. But she said 'You've done everything right it's just bad luck as the cancer is clear cell and just so bloomin aggressive.' So another comment on this, if you have radiotherapy or surgery or anything interventional to one specific area of the body, discuss with your oncologist about still staying on a systemic treatment, especially if you have clear cell, since you are then covering all bases so to speak.

I think the first thought for everyone when you see tumours is 'Get them out of my body' but the concern was how could you shrink a 10cm tumour in the liver with drugs?

Anyway my surgeon recommended another oncologist, this time a clinical oncologist in a new clinic that had recently opened, and he mentioned that they also did some off label drug treatment like immunotherapy, so myself and my brother agreed that we had nothing to lose.

In case anyone isn't clear between the difference, a clinical oncologist handles drugs but also interventional treatments like radiotherapy, radio frequency ablation, chemo embolisation and a medical oncologist is a specialist on drugs.

Before seeing the new oncologist I did more research. It was clear for instance, that chemotherapy was not going to work long term for me and now new research is showing that clear cell ovarian cancer does not really react well to chemotherapy, although I know one lady in a Facebook group I belong to who's been NED (No Evidence of Disease) for 12 years! But for most it comes back within 3 to 5 years, not everyone, as the body is different in each individual, but for the majority. If you are diagnosed at Stage 1 you have a better chance, but that still didn't apply to me, as I have severe spread, although I am confident that I will live over the 5 years which as mentioned seems to be the average mortality rate when you reach stage 4.

I researched firstly into RFA or Radio Frequency Ablation when a hot probe is inserted into the tumour and heated up to a high temperature which then, basically, fries the tumour. To the liver it is just like a little tickle and doesn't do much damage to it, it just leaves scarring. The liver is the only organ in the body that can amazingly regenerate itself and grow back, which is a miracle really. The only catch is that the tumour mustn't be too near to a vital artery or another blood vessel and that the tumour isn't over 4cm. For the 6 tumours in the right lobe of the liver RFA was a possibility for me, but for the 10cm one it was way too big.

I also researched into chemo embolisation, which is for bigger tumours. This is where a line is inserted into the tumour and it is treated with chemotherapy. It can be a stronger dose as it is infused directly into the tumour. So maybe this was also an option to be discussed.

Just to note here that there is now also a fantastic doctor in the US who is able to inject immunotherapy drugs directly into tumours through guided ultrasound and having a lot of success. This is groundbreaking treatment and I hope more doctors will be able to do this in the future.

I was also going to ask about targeted drugs; these are taken orally or by IV infusion depending on the drug, for the antiangiogenic ones, they in brief, stop the blood flow to the tumour so that it shrivels up and dies. However, with my history of blood clots this could be a risk since these type of targeted drugs can also cause blood clots. Targeted drugs are actually a broad description as immunotherapy drugs can also be classed in this genre.

I think when you get to the stage when your liver has 7 tumours in it, the dark thoughts do start and you feel 'God I'll try anything now' to help.

One of my neighbours said that she had gone to school with a very interesting guy who had worked for pharmaceutical companies doing research and had a great understanding of drugs, Dr Robin Bannister. His wife had late stage breast cancer and he wanted, with all his knowledge, to try and cure her, or at least prolong her life. Unfortunately, she passed away in 2017. He set up a private clinic in London called the Care Oncology Clinic and had basically worked on a protocol for off the shelf drugs that were cheap to buy and were found to have some success in keeping cancer tumours stable, or weakening them to make drugs like chemotherapy more effective. I truly believe this is an interesting route to follow, but feel more research needs to be done in this area. Large pharmaceutical companies are reluctant to run any drug trials to test this metabolic approach as these drugs are already in use for other ailments and can be bought off the shelf, so they would be unable to recoup any money from doing drug trials.

I know many people call these companies 'Big Pharma' and are very critical of them, saying they are greedy and just out to make money. Well, everyone has their own opinion on this, but if you think about how many billions of pounds or dollars are spent on testing these drugs to get them safe, effective and available on the market for use, they have to get their money back somehow? If you think of the process....... a Phase 1 drug trial is to test the safety of the drug and its dosage; testing it on between 20 to 100 patients and can take weeks or months. If proven to be safe then the Phase 2 trial moves on to test the efficacy of the drug on different cancers and further evaluate safety, this is tested on less than 200 patients over a time span of 2 years. If it is proven to be effective, then a Phase 3 trial includes a much wider population of patients, up to thousands and compares the new drug against standard treatments taking around 4 years to again test the efficacy. If this is seen to be effective then it gets approval which can take 2 years. It then goes to a Phase 4 trial with hundreds of thousands of patients to further test efficacy and safety which can also take 2 years. So, I think that calculates to be approximately 9 years, plus the original drug research of 4 years and with the preclinical lab and animal trials, you are talking a minimum of 12 years and only 5% of these drugs get approved! – I can't logically criticise them for wanting to recoup some of the cost can you?

Back to Dr Robin Bannister, the 4 drugs recommended are Metformin used for diabetics which lowers the glucose level in the body, statins which are used to lower cholesterol, an antibiotic and a worming tablet.

I spoke personally to Robin after my friend gave me his mobile and then had a consultation with one of the doctors at COC its abbreviation and spent a lot of money on this. However, I did have a query about taking the antibiotic, having had issues with these before with candida in my stomach, but never got a reply and was too tired to chase again, so not particularly impressed. I tried the protocol and spent 500 pounds on these drugs. We have a wonderful pharmacy here in Hong Kong where you can buy most drugs off the shelf, so I was able to get hold of them here. I bought 3 months worth, however wouldn't say that 500 pounds was cheap! I think they are probably cheaper in the UK though.

The Metformin made me vomit continuously, the statins added to my already painful joint pain and the antibiotic gave me candida, as I feared it would and added to an already inflamed bowel and stomach.

Although I'm sure the thinking behind this route is sound it wasn't for me sadly. Luckily, I have a friend following this protocol and could give her all the drugs so they weren't wasted. I know of other ovarian cancer patients that also followed this protocol, but to no avail, so maybe it isn't so effective for ovarian cancer?

There is a fantastic lady who has just written an excellent book looking at all the metabolic pathways for tumour proliferation and has good suggestions on how to block them with off label drugs, but because my immunotherapy is such a new drug and still on drug trial it is difficult to know whether there will be interactions. If it came to the point where I ran out of options for conventional drugs then I would look into using these drugs or also Chinese Medicine which is very powerful.

Digressed a bit! But my next step was to go and visit the new oncologist. One of my dear friends from Cancer Connect came with me to give me support and in fact recorded the conversation for me so I could play it back later.

We had a long discussion on what the next protocol should be. Chemotherapy and radiotherapy clearly hadn't worked and I wondered what options were left for me. There is one targeted drug called Avastin which is FDA approved for use with ovarian cancer but my previous oncologist and also this one were very wary of using it as it can cause blood clots, and as I've had 2 already they both thought the risk was too high. However, my haematology oncologist, which I believe I mentioned before, had told me that once I was taking heparin daily it would be very unlikely I could get a blood clot.

We discussed at length the use of a new immunotherapy drug called Pembrolizumab, or brand name Keytruda, which had about a 30% success rate with ovarian cancer patients, not just clear cell but all types of ovarian cancer. The shortest timeline for it to kick in was a minimum of 3 months and we all felt that there wasn't enough time for this to happen before my liver began to fail. Also, I called my broker on the spot there and then to ask if the immunotherapy was covered by the insurance, but he said no, it was deemed experimental and therefore not covered (it was only FDA approved for melanoma and non-small cell lung cancer at that time) however we could try and put a case together for it.

I also asked about doing another NG Sequencing test to see if the cancer had mutated and if I might have a new genomic mutation that we could target, but the oncologist wasn't very keen on the test.

I also enquired about RFA but most of the tumours were too big, so even if we zapped the small ones it wouldn't get rid of the large ones.

We discussed chemo and knew that although it wasn't effective long term, perhaps it was a chance to shrink the tumours and stop progression to buy me time to have a shot at immunotherapy. So, we decided to go down the chemotherapy route with a different drug called Doxorubicin, or brand name Caelyx, together with Carboplatin, which I had previously. I was naturally a bit reluctant to have it as my ARID1A gene suggests that clear cell ovarian cancer is immune to platinum based therapy, however it needed to be used as it worked as a catalyst for the Doxorubicin, so then this made sense. A lot of drugs are used in combination so that they both work together as dual therapies rather than a one therapy or a monotherapy.

Before having this I needed to have an echo and ECG as Doxorubicin can damage the heart, so it's not good to administer this if you have a heart complaint.

I also found out about a specialist gynaecological consultant in the UK who specialised in ovarian cancer and immunotherapy plus has a lot of knowledge regarding clear cell ovarian cancer. She recommended that I should absolutely try immunotherapy as there had been good success with clear cell ovarian cancer and agreed that chemotherapy was showing to be ineffective long term for clear cell. As second line, she recommended a targeted drug together with chemotherapy. She said she was soon to start a drug trial with Pembrolizumab (Keytruda) a monoclonal anti body, (anti PD1) specifically on clear cell ovarian cancer patients but I would not be eligible. However, that did give me hope that immunotherapy was seriously being considered for clear cell ovarian cancer. She said that most research showed that patients need to stay on the drug for 2 years, then take a break and if it came back within a year go back on the drug for another year.

My heart check came back clear and we began the treatment. Doxorubicin is interesting as it is pink! So, it looks like you're being pumped full of pink grapefruit juice or an exotic cocktail! But as you can imagine it's no fun in reality!

The new clinic was really nice. Because I was too tall for the chemotherapy chairs I was given a VIP room with a bed and TV to watch. So very civilised! Also they had proper infusion machines (rather than a bag of drugs hung on a rail which was what I'd had previously) and flushed my veins through with saline before and after treatment to minimise side effects. It made the whole experience much more palatable.

After 2 cycles we scanned to see what was happening and unfortunately our plan hadn't paid off as the 10cm tumour had grown to 11cm, but some of the smaller ones had reduced in size a bit. Another one had also appeared though, so in total 8 now!!!

The oncologist strongly suggested that I start immunotherapy treatment as I had nothing to lose and so we decided to have my first dose immediately after the consultation. Immunotherapy is worked out so that you have 2mg for every 1kg of body weight and as I am a big girl, both tall and holding a lot of weight from the previous drug treatment, I needed 200mg of the drug. This works out at a cost of 8,200 pounds each treatment, so expensive, but we decided to bite the bullet and do it.

My mum and brother who came to support me for the results took it all in their stride and then mum suddenly piped up and said 'Why can't she have a liver transplant?' The oncologist smiled and then thought about it and said, 'Actually I can refer you to our medical director here a professor, who is a world famous surgeon, and see what he thinks. If anyone can operate then he can!'

The following day we returned to the clinic, myself and my brother and spoke with this professor. He said immediately that he had studied the PET scan results and that he could operate, remove the left lobe of my liver where the 11cm tumour was situated and also another fairly large one. Then on the right lobe he could do RFA to zap the other tumours and it would all be taken out.

The one great thing about having private medical insurance is that you can be in hospital almost immediately after the decision is made! After I got approval from the insurance company, we were ready to go a week later. I was booked into The Adventist hospital a different hospital again from the previous but one where this doctor preferred to operate. I also decided to have a private room again as I knew I was going to be in a lot of discomfort after the operation and wanted my own space.

The Adventist Hospital is the only hospital in Hong Kong that does direct billing for my insurance company, yes! and oh, how much easier to deal with! A guarantee of payment still needs to be arranged, but if costs run over for any reason they can just phone up the insurance company directly and get an extension, rather than me or my broker having to chase around for all the paperwork etc. The last thing you need when you are coming out of hospital after surgery, is to be stressed about all the payment. I will always choose The Adventist Hospital for treatment now where possible.

Basically, the surgeon told me that I would be cut down the centre of my chest and then round across my right-hand side, across my liver so forming an L shape. He would remove my left lobe and then perform RFA while I was opened up.

I got all unpacked and settled in my room only to be told by the nurse that it was such a major operation that I might need to go to ICU after surgery for observation. Therefore I may not be coming back to the same room. I did get a bit emotional then and say 'Why can't we keep the room. I've unpacked now can't we just pay for it and then when I move out of ICU I can come back to it'. But oh no, that seemed too difficult as they could offer the room to another patient and then I would need to take pot luck once I came out of the ICU. I wasn't happy and just wanted to come back to my room and recover. Actually, I hadn't realised how major the surgery was but I did go straight back to my room as I'm a tough cookie and didn't need to go to ICU. The fact that I am quite a big girl helps me in that way I believe, as a strong body.

I was nervous on the day of surgery but it all went well. I remember waking up in the corner of the operating theatre in excruciating pain with a nurse standing over me, and saying 'God it hurts', and her saying 'I know you should see the size of the piece of liver we took out!' And I'm thinking 'Yes, I can bloody feel it!'

But then must have zonked out again as next time I woke up I was in my room with my sister in law standing over me. So nice to see a familiar face; with me saying 'Ouch, ouch it hurts' and the nurse saying 'I'm pumping drugs into you as quick as I can'. The nurse doing this and the nurse who looked after me for most of my stay was a lovely Scottish nurse, so nice to have an expat nurse looking after you, who understood the dry humour, all the little nuances of being an expat in a foreign country she made it all bearable.

I also had a catheter in my bladder which I've had for both other abdomen surgeries, but thought I would mention it here. Love the catheter, as you don't need to struggle up to use the loo all the time, as I said before, I don't do well with bedpans. Although there is risk of infection the longer you keep it in, I always try to squeeze one more day as it is so much easier!

On my second day out of surgery, a very bubbly physiotherapist came in and said 'I'm here to ensure that you inflate your lungs properly and get moving.' I wasn't told I would have a physio to come in and see me and was really grouchy saying 'Who said you should come here, I don't want a physio, I've not had one before from last surgeries'. 'Well, you have a partially collapsed lung on your X-Ray, so you need to get this moving.' As you can imagine, straight after surgery, with a whacking big wound down from my chest, it was really, really, painful to try and take big breaths! But I tried my best. My oxygen levels had dropped a bit too, I guess, from the collapsed lung, so I had to have oxygen pumped in for a while also.

The physio was actually very good and used to come in and see me morning and night, had trained and lived in Australia and did become someone that I got on with really well. The Adventist has a circular arrangement for its floors so you could walk round in a circle and do one circuit. As I got stronger I could do several circuits.

I have to say I was in considerable pain for quite a few days and then the wound obviously started to heal and I found this quite uncomfortable as my skin seemed to be stretched. When the dressing came off later I realised that I was stapled all the way up on my wound, so I can understand my discomfort now!

The Adventist is a wonderful hospital except it only supplies vegetarian food. It is partly for religious reasons and also for health reasons. I was only taking liquids for quite a while until my bowels moved and then it was all OK. I can really truly only eat so many floppy mushrooms though!

Luckily one of our dear friends was regularly bringing up her husband for physio, so she used to bring me lovely roast chicken to keep me going! Also, I had visits daily from my cancer support group friends so always had company and snacks brought in. In fact, The Adventist does provide a fast food delivery number if you want to order in other food like MEAT! So they obviously realised the need for patients to have that choice. If god wanted us to be vegetarians then he would have made us like cows or something! Just my opinion, but we are omnivores and so feel our bodies need an all-round diet. As I said previously, just my opinion mind, I'm sure many people would disagree. If we get on to animal farming and the impact on the environment then that is altogether a different matter.

I spent 10 days in hospital and gradually recovered. The gas in the bowels thing was very painful again, but as mentioned before I know now to request an enema and that would get things moving!

When I got all my discharge papers I saw that it read that I'd had my gall bladder removed too. When I challenged my surgeon, he said 'Oh yes, we took that out also, but I didn't think you'd be interested in those technical things.' Yeah right! I think I'd like to know if my gall bladder was removed! But actually, it's not a problem, just means that I need to avoid fat, but I do that anyway so even more incentive really. I also saw a picture of the huge tumour they removed. I always thought cancer tumours were black nasty things, as that's what they show up as on scans. But actually, they look like those natural Greek sponges you can buy, but white, or a white piece of coral. Lots of holes in it. Nasty things anyway and glad they were out!

It was quite uncomfortable getting home to Discovery Bay as it allows no cars! So we had to order an ambulance to take me home. It was a charity run one not the large St John's ambulance that just glides along, so I felt every bump! Did take the pain meds, but they kicked in too late!

We have since moved for many reasons, but one for sure was the transport issue.

Once at home I needed to recover fully, but it didn't take too long and my surgeon was able to remove my staples, which did become very uncomfortable as they were unable to stretch with the skin as it healed over. So I was glad to get them out to be honest! I did need to use the wheel chair for a while though, and it was a bit of a challenge getting in and out of bed. When I first went home we had the foldable bed we used for guests in the sitting room, with our helper sleeping on the sofa. As it was low it was the only bed I could get up from when I needed to go to the loo in the night. One big advantage of living in Hong Kong is the luxury of having a helper. They are usually Filipino, which ours is. We have been through a few for various reasons, but our current one is part of the family, is a trained nurse and has done an elderly care course so she is a godsend. My big brother pays her salary since he travels so much with his job, he wants to ensure that myself and my mum have someone to look after us. It's really good of him to do that.

A month after surgery we did a CT scan just to check that the liver was healing well and growing back, but noticed another black shadow on my liver! This could have been scarring my oncologist said, but my surgeon thought it was probably another tumour that had somehow been missed. No one's fault by the way, just the way it is. We probably should have done a PET/CT combined, which is what I always have now as the CT, which uses a dye, can see the makeup of all the tumours, which is very helpful, but doesn't show if they are glowing or not (i.e. active) which the PET scan does.

So the choice was to leave it and see if the immunotherapy worked or do RFA extraneously this time. 'Nooo' says I, 'Get it out, don't take any risks,' it was the best decision in the end as the immunotherapy took ages to kick in later.

I can report also that the none of the tumours that had RFA treatment have recurred, so I do feel it is an effective treatment.

I thought I would have had a general anaesthetic for the RFA and be put to sleep but, oh no, had to be awake to breathe in at the right time to make it more effective.

I was really, really nervous when the day came to have this done, as I really didn't know what was going to happen and more importantly how much pain I would feel. I remember Crane having had this done and saying it was very painful, so I was thinking, yikes! However, how can anything be more painful than having half your liver removed, right?

On the day of the operation I wasn't allowed to eat for 8 hours before. After changing into the operating gown, I lay on the operating table and the radiology consultant, a fantastic man, (I need to say that this was done at my oncology clinic downstairs in the radiotherapy department as an outpatient, where I also have my PET/CT scans done) performed the procedure. An anaesthetist was on hand so, I had a local anaesthetic on the skin and then the probe is put into the liver, that did hurt as I felt a prick, but over in a second. Then the surgeon started to heat up the probe, all done by guided ultrasound and I could see it happening on the screen! And basically, the probe gradually fries the tumour. I was then asked to breathe in and out at intervals. As the probe heated up I felt like I had a very bad heartburn and that's when the anaesthetist pumped in the strong local anaesthetic so I couldn't feel anything, but could watch the tumour gradually being frazzled on the ultrasound screen. It reminds me of one of the 'Carry On' Films I forget which, with the mad Kenneth Williams, turning ladies his side kick Oddbod has kidnapped, into shop mannequins. I recall him saying in a mad voice 'Are we Frying Tonight!!!'. 'Carry On Screaming' I think it was.......

All over in about 20 minutes if that. I was then wheeled next door to recover. This, to be honest, is the most uncomfortable bit, as the strong local anaesthesia wears off you feel like you have incredible indigestion, heart burn, for an hour or so. Pain relief didn't kick in quick enough, so I had to lie there in real discomfort for about an hour. After an hour, the pain subsided and I could eat some soup and then after about 5 hours I was allowed to go home.

Unfortunately, the black rainstorm warning was raised, which means no one is supposed to go out, but we managed to thankfully, get a taxi from the regular company I used to use, especially when I said I'd come out of surgery, so they were very accommodating. I think I paid something like HK$20 extra but no big deal.

I just had to rest when I got home, but no long-lasting effects really, up the next day, removed the plaster over the small hole and off back to enjoy the day.

We then decided to carry on with the immunotherapy as we knew it was pointless doing more chemotherapy.

However, the reality suddenly hit us that this treatment was going to cost us 8,200 pounds (HK$82,000) every 3 weeks and could potentially be needed for up to 2 years, in total something like 36 treatments. I got the oncology consultant in London to write a letter to the insurance company, and also my current oncologist, to say that it was obvious that chemotherapy and radiotherapy had been ineffective and pleaded with my broker to negotiate that the insurance covered the treatment. But the insurance was denied, as the immunotherapy drug Pembrolizumab (Keytruda) just wasn't FDA approved for ovarian cancer and deemed experimental. Very few drugs are approved for use with ovarian cancer, it's always breast cancer out of the hormonal cancers that gets the most funding, despite as mentioned ovarian cancer having the much higher mortality rate globally, around 60%, as opposed to 10% for breast cancer.

It all seemed like doom and gloom, and then I said right 'OK I'm going to swallow my pride, it's a bit embarrassing but I'm going to ask friends, family, colleagues to help and try and fundraise.' I was totally, totally blown away by the generosity of everyone! It seemed that they had all wanted to help, but didn't know how and this was a way of saving my life!

Many people gave donations, really generous donations like the cost of one treatment! And others did some fabulous fundraising! Making Christmas chutneys and chocolates, holding Christmas fairs, head shaving, junk trips with an auction, tandem paraglides! Everything! It was not only the money, it was just the love that I felt coming from everyone which just kept me going so much! I also sold off clothes, jewellery, books and made some dogs treats, as I knew in Discovery Bay everyone loved their dogs. Just anything to raise money.

One of my dear friends came up with the name for the fundraising campaign, 'Hilary's Hope Fund'. It is my dream that after I have published this book I will be able to set up a registered charity with this name, to support funding for ovarian cancer research, or other ovarian cancer patients with funding for treatment. At the time of the fundraising for my personal treatment, many companies said they would have donated had Hilary's Hope Fund been a registered charity. Setting up a charity, like everything, costs money, so I hope the sales from this book will also enable me to do that, while also being able to give a percentage to ovarian cancer research.

In the end, everyone raised 50,000 pounds (HK$500,000) which funded 5 treatments initially which was amazing. I wanted to join in the tandem paraglide group, but we had to walk up a steep hill and a bit of a hike to reach the top and it was just so hot that I couldn't make it. I was so upset, but saw the video afterwards, which was fabulous. My dear friend Anne-Marie was actually terrified of heights, but did that for me. What a wonderful friend. My other closest and dearest friend Sara walked back down with me. I was so grateful for her support and the paragliding instructor drove us to some random shopping centre in the middle of nowhere, so we decided to go back to Discovery Bay and relax on her boat. Had we thought of it there was a very nice Grand Hyatt hotel where we could have waited for the group, but forgot it was there so missed them.

If anyone is struggling for treatment money I would one hundred percent suggest fundraising, as people want to help but don't know how sometimes!

So I had the stress of funding the treatment taken away and began my 3 weekly sessions.

In the appendix, it advises on how all the drugs work, so do please use that as a reference to explain how Keytruda works.

The first thing anyone will find when on immunotherapy is the incredible, incredible fatigue. No matter how much you sleep you still feel like you've only had about 2 hours' sleep! This is because of the inflammation. The body constantly thinks it's recovering from flu so is putting all its energy into attacking the virus. Thinking positively, this is good, as it means that the drug is doing its job. I also suffered from terrible hot flushes. This may have been related to having had my ovaries removed, but I could be happily chatting to someone and then I could, literally, be feeling it move up my body into my face and just started sweating. Then, after only a few minutes, I could feel it all slowly progressing back down the body and finished. I'm sure many women experience the same thing going through menopause and I can really sympathise! The only thing that helped me was Sage supplements recommended by the oncologist in Bath. Evening Primrose Oil did nothing, Black Cohosh did nothing, but Sage did work. The thing is, that I discovered Sage can also inflame the body though, so stopped taking the supplements as more inflammation was not what I needed! I have since decided that the hot flushes are actually something to do with the immune system working, as every time I had a treatment I would struggle with hot flushes, but now very rarely have them since my tumour burden is so low it doesn't need to work as hard.

Life went on, treatment every 3 weeks parting with HK$82,000 each time was painful! But that's what it cost so it was what it was!

I felt fine really, apart from the fatigue and for about a week I got this awful vertigo, which had me in tears! Even lying down it felt like the walls were closing in and everything kept flipping over and when I tried to sit up it was dreadful, everything was just spinning. I couldn't even make it to the loo and remember my mother and our helper getting my mum's frame that she had over her loo, with a bucket underneath and both of them heaving me up on to the make shift commode to have a wee, which I was desperate for. The sheer humiliation, although it was only my mother and our helper, was just so awful that I cried so much. Like so many times with the disease, it's the loss of control of your body that I frequently just can't handle.

After that episode we enjoyed life and I carried on working and just felt so blessed to be on a treatment that could potentially cure me or at least keep my disease stable.

I remember having a wonderful Christmas with family and friends and putting the PET scan, which I was about to have, in the background. I think this is the mentally challenging thing for me, my cancer has never given me any pain, so it has always lulled me into a false sense of security almost. You always feel not that bad and happily carry on with life forgetting to some extent that you even have cancer and then boom! Along come the PET scan results and the stress and worry begin again.

Chapter Five

The Fourth Recurrence

When we went for the PET scan results I felt so well that I was convinced that the immunotherapy was working. My cancer marker was low and I was feeling really good, but again, how wrong could I be?

My mum and my brother accompanied me and by sheer luck, (the universe was looking out for me that day) my regular oncologist was on holiday for Christmas and I saw a lady oncologist that day. She is now my oncologist as we all looked at each other when I got my results and we said 'We like you, please can we change to you now as my oncologist.' I can only say that she is the best! I would not be in the shape I am in now without her knowledge and also the willingness to work as a team. Many of my friends from my cancer group often consult with her now for advice, as she is amazing at looking into what drives the tumour to grow, what mutations it has, really on the ball.

She had the task of dropping the bombshell too, which was devastating. I was not looking at stability or remission, the cancer had spread again, this time to 22 tumours. More in my liver, in my lungs, one in my left hip bone and in my lymph nodes. All I could think about was, 'Oh god, oh god, I'm definitely not coming back from this. God that could have been my last Christmas. Panic, panic'.

The oncologist said that she could have considered inflammation, as immunotherapy can cause what is called pseudo progression when you see progression of what you think are malignant tumours, but they are actually tumours caused by inflammation. For instance, if you had a scan when you had a bad cough from a cold, you would find that you had tumours in your lungs caused by inflammation.

However, as the tumours were over 25% spread, then this was actually benchmarked in the clinical profession as cancer progression or hyper progression.

Immediately, I asked if we could do another NG Sequencing test to see if the tumours had mutated and she said 'Yes! Absolutely' (definitely my kind of oncologist) and she suggested that we add chemo and another targeted drug into the mix. She suggested Abraxane, which is a more modern version of Paclitaxol. I wasn't too keen as this is what had started off my DVT, but she decided to administer it weekly on a lower dose to save the harder hit on the body. For the other drug my oncologist decided to put me on Pazopanib (brand name Votrient) as she had recently read research that clear cell ovarian cancer was now showing some characteristics similar to clear cell renal cancer and immunotherapy was being used with a targeted drug, a tyrosine kinase inhibitor which was Votrient. So, despite my blood clot risk she wanted to try this together with the chemo and the immunotherapy. I was injecting heparin daily into my leg so there was little chance of a blood clot anyway now.

This drug also wasn't FDA approved for use with ovarian cancer, but the insurance didn't quibble at all on this and approved it!

It was good news that clear cell ovarian cancer was now being associated with clear cell renal cancer as it was going to hopefully open up a much wider group of cancer patients and therefore access to more drugs. The drugs that are FDA approved for use with ovarian cancer are few and far between so anything that would help with this was a real plus.

So I took the Votrient, 400 mg, 2 tablets a day for a week after immunotherapy and then 600mg 3 tablets a day together until the next immunotherapy treatment plus the chemo weekly. The Votrient at that time had few side effects, although on a bad day could cause diarrhoea and high blood pressure. And my hair started to go silver grey. This was because this drug blocks the VEGFR in the metabolism. My hair is almost all pure white now, including eye brows and body hair, a bit weird, but definitely on trend. My hairdresser keeps telling me that customers pay good money to have their hair my colour! So, there you go! Unintentionally trendy!!

The insurance wouldn't fund my NG Sequencing test, but my brother and sister in law kindly donated the cost to me as part of my fundraising campaign. The sample was used from my previous liver surgery.

So off we went on the chemo and Votrient. I hated the chemo as always and went through all the usual side effects. Constipation, diarrhoea, numbness in the fingers and toes, my hair started to fall out – all the usual stuff! I'm going to skim through the chemo and Votrient bit as nothing much different to say. The NG Sequencing test came back with an additional mutation HER2, so this was something else we could work with. There are some good drugs that are FDA approved for use with breast cancer, Everolimus and Tesirolimus, MTor inhibitors that target the PTEN metabolic pathway that have had success with ovarian cancer, so these were being considered as the next drugs. The next scan in March 2017 looked really good, the tumours had started to regress, the ones in the lungs and liver had all but disappeared, plus the one in the hip bone and all looked positive as down to 12 tumours. My oncologist said there wouldn't have been such a good result had we not had the immunotherapy as well, so finally perhaps it was kicking in. On heavily pre-treated patients like myself, who have gone down so many lines of chemotherapy, it is said that it takes the immunotherapy a lot longer to kick in and re-programme the T-cells.

Around this time I'd started getting funny things happening with my heart. It would suddenly speed up uncontrollably, and it was very scary when it did that. It also started jumping around quite a lot. So my oncologist recommended that I go to see a cardiologist, which I did, and he referred me to The Hong Kong Sanatorium hospital to be fitted with a halter monitor to follow my heart beats over a 24 hour period. This was pretty straightforward, I just needed to make a note of the time and what happened when I felt the heart jumping around. When I went back to the cardiologist he explained that I had arrhythmia, which could have possibly been caused by the Caelyx (Doxorubicin) chemotherapy, as I think I mentioned before that one of the side effects is heart damage. He said it wasn't too serious, but prescribed me a drug called Concor which slows down the heart beat and therefore prevents it from speeding up.

Also at this time I was suffering from very uncomfortable constipation. We discovered that the Kytril, my anti-nausea drug was causing this. I think I have mentioned that if you get constipated it doesn't really matter how much fruit, fibre, drugs like Senakot, Lactulose you use, once the bowel has stopped then my gastroenterologist advised glycerin suppositories were the solution. Have to agree that they work every time. So we stopped the Kytril and by doing that I had no problems whatsoever with constipation. Unfortunately, with constipation came haemorrhoids. I had small ones from doing a lot of horse riding when I was young, sitting on hard riding saddles, and these would flare up if occasionally I sat on a hard seat for too long. But since having really bad constipation frequently, they had become quite large and really caused a lot of bleeding when they flared up.

In the next scan in July 2017 we were down to 8 tumours, however 2 more were back in the liver and some of the lymph nodes, particularly one in my porta hepatis lymph node which kept changing in SUV level, had shot up to 21 in activity, so very aggressive. The scan in March had been really good but just didn't bring stability. I had also got a very bad cold during the chemo this time and my white bloods had dropped and we couldn't get them back up so I had to inject white blood cell boosters to bump them back up every 3 days in the first week of treatment. I missed a fair amount of the chemo due to my cold and the state of the white blood cells so in the end my oncologist decided to stop it and continue just with the immunotherapy and the Votrient, since they had been the main players in the last month or so in terms of higher dosage.

As soon as we had more tumours back in the liver my first thought was 'Get rid of them, get rid of them,' but my oncologist said that it just wasn't worth doing RFA on them since I had active disease elsewhere. She said she would only do it if we were left with tumours in the liver and the disease was stable or gone everywhere else. This was fair enough, but I still wasn't happy about it as my one fear was getting tumours back in the liver, as you only have one and mine was already compromised. I then had an idea and suggested, from my experience with the RFA, 'Why don't we do an ultrasound as an interim between PET scans?' You can see the tumours in and around the liver (that's how they get guided for the RFA) so we could at least see if they were getting bigger, even if we couldn't see their SUV activity and we could also see if there were more appearing. So we compromised on this and I now regularly have an interim ultrasound between PET scans.

When we had regression and things looked really positive and it seemed like the immunotherapy was working, we just didn't know what to do about the money side. Usually patients who have a good response stay on Keytruda for 2 years, this meant we needed to find around HK$3M about GBP300,000. The fundraising was so good but finding that kind of money we needed some kind of miracle. In the end I decided to bite the bullet and speak with my boss and just put it bluntly. 'We are talking about whether I live or die here and the insurance just wouldn't cover the immunotherapy treatment as although it is approved for use with melanoma and small cell lung cancer, it's still seen as experimental for ovarian cancer. However if I have chemotherapy it will be roughly the same cost, as I will need drugs to counterbalance the side effects so it just seems so unfair.' My boss spoke with our HR department and they in turn spoke to the company broker, who in turn spoke with the insurance company and in the end, after costs were supplied for the cost of chemo against immunotherapy, which balanced out as the same, then the insurance company saw that it made sense and agreed to fund the immunotherapy. However, in November 2017 the FDA approved the use of immunotherapy on all solid tumours with micro satellite status high and tumour mutation burden high so actually our request wasn't 'way out there' in the end. I am actually MSI Stable and TMB Low! But the company insurance is covering all the treatment. I am really, really blessed to love my job and love my company, to work for senior management who care so much about the wellbeing of their staff is just so wonderful. I can work from home if the side effects are bad some days but I work hard from home or probably work even harder as no distracting conversations!

I know not all companies are like that, so I am thankful for how much they care. It's taken so much worry and pressure off me, knowing that I don't need to worry about the money side and can just concentrate on healing myself and enjoying my work.

I know drug companies have to charge a lot of money for their drugs due to the cost of the drugs trials, but it excludes so many cancer patients who can only get access to these drugs via clinical trials as it's too late for them by the time the drugs are FDA approved for use with their type of cancer. When it's about whether you have the chance to live for many years or die it's a cruel position for so many people and their families to face. The sad fact of life is that so many cancer patients do find themselves in this position. I have heard of patients being able to get access to drugs that are not approved for use with their cancer on compassionate use, i.e. they will be dead before they can officially use this drug for their type of cancer, but have never really considered asking this question. If this is really the case then the drug companies are not all bad.

As mentioned before, you now start thinking I'll try anything to stop this damn cancer, so I consulted with a lovely lady in the UK who had previously, been a chemotherapy nurse and had noticed that patients who followed an integrative treatment fared better than patients who just followed a conventional method of treatment. I had a call with her and she suggested some interesting alternative therapies, one being cannabis oil. Once again, hugely expensive; it cost me about 700 pounds for all the drugs, but I was prepared to give it a go. Unfortunately, the cannabis oil interacted with my targeted drug and just really stressed me out, not making me high, but really making me anxious and stressed. Recent research has also now suggested that cannabis oil can interfere with immunotherapy to make it less effective. Therefore, although all these people mean well they are not your oncologist and they don't really know about all the interactions with the newer drugs like immunotherapy, so you must be really careful about using alternative therapies. Unless you really know what you are doing it can be quite dangerous.

However, she did advise that having an oxygenator would be excellent, as cancer isn't a fan of oxygen and this could help in the healing process. An oxygenator doesn't pump out oxygen, as it is dangerous to use pure oxygen, but it cleans the air through the processing in the machine, so you get a good blast of clean air into your lungs daily. I rented one on a monthly basis from a local supplier, Celki Air, which did really work and reduced the fatigue and made me feel more energetic and better for using it. I don't now, as I am trying to use a CPAP machine at night due to Sleep Apnea (will come on to that later) so saw no benefit in having air pumped into me by 2 different sources.

At this time, I had seen little publicity or information about ovarian cancer in Hong Kong and decided that it was time that the profile was raised more. I knew that March was ovarian cancer month in the UK and so e-mailed the 'South China Morning Post,' who are the biggest English speaking national newspaper in Hong Kong, with my story to see what happened. Immediately, a reporter, a lovely American guy, contacted me. He was a freelance journalist who wrote many of the health features in the SCMP and asked to come and do an interview with me and he would also bring a photographer. He was a lovely guy and wrote a very good one page feature. One of the main messages I wanted to get across is for women to notice their symptoms and to get checked out. They are, as I have previously mentioned, so easy to miss. I didn't have much communication back from this article, but hope the readers did take note. It did also mention how friends, family who interact/care for people with cancer can communicate better, as we didn't cause this disease, we are not lepers, cancer is not catching. We are people with feelings, hopes, dreams just like anyone else and we need your support, not to be shunned as some alien, or for our illness to be ignored. One of the phrases I hate the most and I think most cancer patients will say the same is 'Keep Fighting', 'Get Well Soon', 'Stay Positive' – well, what do you think we are doing? of course we are fighting, at stage 4 we aren't going to 'Get Well Soon' and we are in fact only going to get worse over time and eventually sadly die and yes of course we will stay positive! Perhaps that's why some people won't talk to you for fear of saying the wrong thing. But it's horrible being ignored as if you are some second-class citizen just because you have a chronic illness.

I have since done some Press interviews which I will discuss later where I did get a lot of feedback from patients particularly with clear cell ovarian cancer (which of course has the highest percentage of patients in Asia) so this was great and I was able to support with a lot of information to make a difference.

A few months in to taking the Votrient, I started to get really bad diarrhoea. My oncologist was worried it was colitis (inflammation) caused by the immunotherapy, and was almost ready to send me for a colonoscopy to investigate this. My cancer marker had started climbing into the 20's and it was very worrying. I had a PET/CT to see what was happening, but things weren't too bad, more activity in the liver and another few lymph nodes had appeared as being active.

Since my stools were yellow I wondered if it was the Curcumin I was taking that might be doing something, or the other supplements. I started to experiment and finally discovered that it was the Berberine that was causing the diarrhoea! I stopped this immediately and blow me down the diarrhoea stopped, and on the scan I had 3 months later all the tumours were regressing once again! Basically, I had been pooing out the Votrient with the diarrhoea. I mentioned this beforehand, I will mention this again here. BE VERY careful when taking supplements with cancer drugs, as they do interact and can affect the efficacy, and also cause other factors like the Berberine and my diarrhoea. I took Curcumin for quite a long time on blood thinners, plus Resveratrol (you find this in red wine), until I realised that they naturally thin blood, so very dangerous to take these with blood thinners!! Once I came off the Berberine and the diarrhoea improved, my cancer marker started to drop again.

Just to add in here, rightly or wrongly, I also use toothpaste without fluoride, deodorant without aluminum or parabens, natural soap, natural shower gel and also shampoo, conditioner and face moisturiser which are paraben free and all natural. I also found a talcum powder which is made from grapefruit seed and tea tree oil – so whether this all makes a difference or not I don't know, but I feel I am giving my body the best chance to avoid toxins, so I know in my heart I've done the best that I can to give my body a chance to heal itself.

Around March 2018 I caught a particularly horrible fluey virus from a colleague at work and unfortunately my mum also got it. It knocked us back. For six weeks we were really poorly and mum even had suspected pneumonia, but antibiotics helped her hugely. It felt like a horrible set back and I was inconsistent in taking the Votrient at that time. I was in fact incredibly angry that I had been doing really well and that my colleague selfishly had come into the office and passed on the virus. He happily recovered quite quickly, while both myself and mum were terribly ill. I think again a word of advice is to 'mask up' and wear a surgical face mask when out and about if there are bugs going around. People with a normal, strong, healthy, immune system just don't think about the fact that they are feeling a bit unwell and come into work, while the germs they are carrying can hit someone with a compromised immune system very hard. A message to you all! If you are sick then stay at home and keep your germs to yourself! All cancer patients going through treatment don't want them thank you very much!!! And the worst place to visit is a hospital! As that is full of bugs! So at all costs I try to avoid hospitals if possible!

At this point I just want to introduce my oncology nurse Tracy. The cancer treatment is often grueling and you don't feel well a lot of the time, plus dealing with insurance companies is also challenging. To have a really fantastic nurse, as I have with Tracy, for me is vital. Her knowledge of cancer treatment, her bright personality (even when I know she isn't always feeling well), her generous and genuine spirit keep me going. She is always on call via What's App, incredibly hard working and for me, I think the oncology nurses are sometimes forgotten. So this is my dedication to them. Thank you so much for getting me through all the dark days and for me to know that I always have someone that I can call on for support. I would like to clone Tracy though, as she is exceptional and irreplaceable!

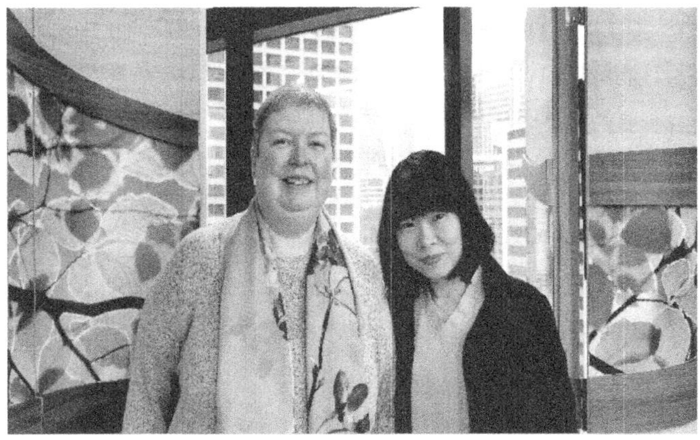

You will probably notice in the picture with Tracy that I had put on a lot of weight. Having lost it when I came off the steroids, this time it was caused by the immunotherapy. It is documented that it can eventually affect the endocrine system and you can also get water retention. Many patients on immunotherapy suffer from lymphoedema (swelling up of legs and ankles). I am at a consistent weight now of 108kg's, it never goes up or down, whether I exercise or not or cut down on food or not, or even have diarrhoea or vomiting, I just stay at the same weight.

During 2018 I continued with the treatment. On some scans we might see another tumour, but my oncologist said 'Don't worry I don't t think we need to do anything. It is probably pseudo progression' i.e. inflammation, and sure enough it was, as on the next scan it would be gone.

I often had issues with my haemorrhoids getting inflamed after treatment, so I knew that I had mild inflammation in the body just after treatment. I have seen some posts in my Facebook groups with cancer patients panicking when they see a toilet bowl full of blood, or the toilet paper soaked in blood. But for me I knew if it was fresh blood and I could feel the haemorrhoid pop then I knew this was nothing to worry about. A spot of Anusol cream for a few days and that would do the trick. I did start taking a cushion to the office though, so I could sit on something soft. My oncologist has since given me a great drug called Daflon which stops the blood building up in the haemorrhoid, which has been very effective in stopping the bleeding, as if it's heavy you can get a bit anaemic.

The only tumour that just didn't seem to be reducing in activity was the one in the porta hepatis lymph node, which just kept jumping in activity from 21 to 16 to 18 to 20, so my oncologist decided to do a biopsy at the end of 2018 to see if this specific tumour had mutated. Since it was in a difficult location the only way to do a biopsy was to do something similar to an endoscopy, where the surgeon went in through the oesophagus and fed through to the tumour that way.

Whilst we decided to do this my oncologist also said 'Why don't we do a colonoscopy too, just to check the bowel is in good shape'. This was a good idea as the prep was the same.

For anyone who has had a gastroscopy or a colonoscopy you will know that you have to restrict your diet, gradually moving in to eating soft food, and then soup and then on the night before the procedure you are given a drink to clear your system. Ghastly thing, as you then just go to the loo constantly to clear your bowels. If you ever have this prepare to have a sleepless night, and if you stay in overnight in the hospital, and if you are in a shared ward, make sure you have a bed pan handy as when you have to go, you have to go, and if someone is in the loo things can get messy! You can do all this at home though, and then come in for the procedure on the day, but this is normally carried out pretty early in hospitals here, like 7.30 to 8am, so that you can recover and eat afterwards, and be out by the afternoon on the same day.

I did stay in, but had a private room so no issues having 100% access to the toilet!

There are only a few doctors in Hong Kong who can do the biopsy procedure I was having, as it is very specialised, but I was lucky to have a good one.

When we were done, he showed me the pot with the tissue specimens in and these were sent off to Foundation One in Boston for my third NG Sequencing test.

About this time I received a note from the women's university association that myself and mum belong to in UK, saying that there was an international poetry competition from a publisher in Hong Kong, Proverse publishing, asking for poems to be submitted. For some reason I just knew that I wanted to write a poem about my mum, and how she has kept me going through this journey from start to finish. I wrote the poem as mentioned previously, 'A Mothers Love', featured at the front of this book in honour of her. I didn't need to change it at all, it just came out straight from deep inside me in one go. When I read it out to mum it brought a tear to her eye and being a Yorkshire lass she rarely shows too much emotion, but she said that it really touched her. Of course, I didn't expect to win, but it was nice when I was told that the poem had been included in 'Mingled Voices 3,' the Proverse prize poetry book for the year 2018. So at this point I must include a picture of my mum and myself from Christmas 2018.

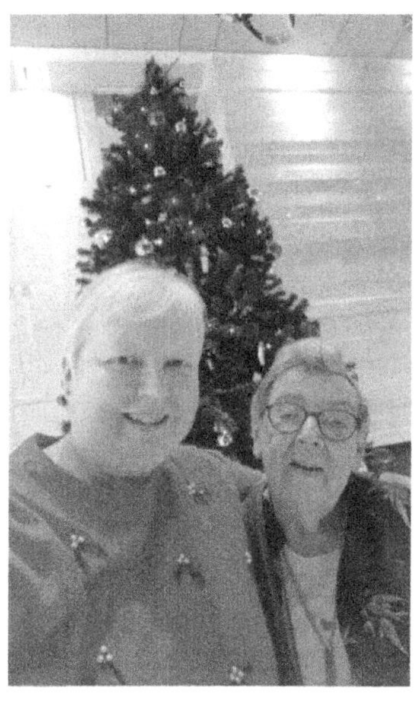

Back to the biopsy! After a few weeks we got the test back and it showed yes, the tumour had an additional mutation, the KRAS mutation. My oncologist said, 'Oh dear that's another nasty and there aren't drugs that can target that specific mutation yet'. Although there isn't a specific drug, down that particular metabolic pathway you have the RAS mutation, the RAF, the MEK and the MAPF there are several drugs that target the MEK and since this is closer to the tumour nucleus than the RAS mutation, by blocking the MEK, the drugs can block the RAS getting to the nucleus. There seem to be several mutations which are drivers for tumour proliferation, TP53 and RAS being two of them. The other mutations I have are less aggressive in terms of this and so can be stabilised better. Luckily I don't have TP53 too! I think the KRAS is enough to cope with!

Hopefully, the diagram below explains my metabolic pathways. The Votrient, being a TKI sort of targets the outside of the tumour so covers all pathways.

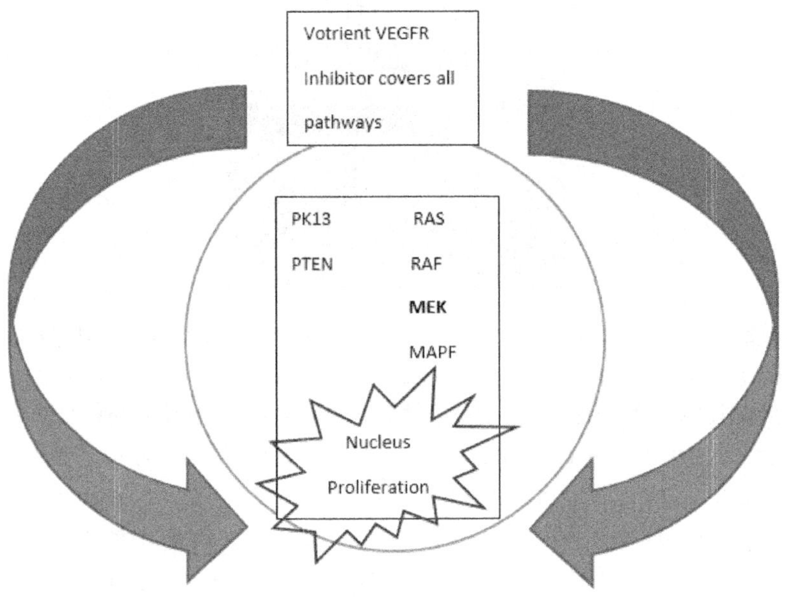

But as it stood, she thought it best to continue on our current regime, since the last scan had shown that the porta hepatis lymph node had reduced to 8 in SUV activity, so this meant that finally, the current drug regime could be working. Also treatments tend to be much quicker to take effect in the larger organs like the liver and lungs, which have lots of blood vessels, and are much slower to reach the lymph nodes to make a difference.

I know pretty much everyone says exercise is good for the system, but I would say in moderation for cancer patients. Pro-Lactin, one of the hormones that is produced by exercise, is also documented as encouraging tumour growth for KRAS mutations, so this is something that I absolutely did not want. When I do very strenuous exercise in the gym, I am so tired that I have to come back and go to bed! That defeats the object really! For me anyway exercise in moderation is the name of the game.

Around this time I also had a bone density scan, as evidence shows that long term use on heparin can cause osteoporosis. The scan came back OK, except in my left hip I was showing signs of osteopenia, the stage before osteoporosis, so we have to keep an eye on this. Eating more calcium enriched foods are excellent and since I don't have anything with dairy, then food like boney fish, i.e. Sardines were good. Also putting the pressure of a heavy weight bearing load would help on it, so lifting a light weight in the gym in my left hand or just a heavy litre bottle of water a day would work. I will have another scan this year just to check how it is all going. My oncologist didn't recommend a calcium supplement as she believed I got enough from food and some of the other supplements I was taking. I was watching a very interesting episode of

'Trust Me I'm A Doctor', presented by Dr Michael Mosely. I always enjoy the tests and experiments they do on the show. This episode was about supplements and the conclusion seemed to be that we do actually get enough supplements from our food and there isn't really an actual need to take additional ones, unless, I guess, it's something very specific.

It was around this time also, that I had a bit of a blood pressure scare. One of the side effects of Votrient is hypertension, so I measure my blood pressure morning and night. It's key to invest in a good blood pressure monitor to ensure you get an accurate reading. For some reason one evening my blood pressure suddenly started to rise and at its highest read 205/113. I felt pretty giddy and knew it was time to take myself off to hospital. Luckily, we have a public hospital right next to our home, which was convenient, although from the experience that I had there I know in future to go to the nearest private hospital. The triage nurse did take my blood pressure immediately, I didn't have to wait and was shown straight through to see a doctor. I had also called my oncologist, it was about midnight by that time, but if she can, she will always answer, how good is that? They recommended a drug called Norvasc to bring the blood pressure down, so I was given this immediately. The blood pressure didn't lower after an hour, so I was given more tablets. It still didn't lower so they wanted to admit me. Public hospitals in Hong Kong are very overcrowded, more than the NHS, so I really didn't want this. They put me in a sort of holding bay instead. The blood pressure cuff they kept using was so small that it squeezed my arm so tight or ripped off, that I found it useless to be honest. There was no way my blood pressure would lower in this kind of environment. So at 4am I checked myself out. Then the following day after little sleep I went to see my oncologist, who also gave me Norvasc and that seemed to work. Apparently, so my oncologist says, the public hospitals can get a different version of the drug which isn't so effective, so that's probably why it didn't work. Lesson learnt. If you have private medical insurance, or even if you don't but can afford it, then go to a private hospital, as the drugs, care etc are sad to say much better. I know sometimes people don't have a choice, and as always we all wish like any country, that the government is able to use more of their funds towards health care.

On my next scan it showed that the SUV activity in the porta hepatis lymph node had dropped right down to 2.54 so almost inactive. For lymph nodes they need to drop down to about 2 to be considered benign. All other disease was virtually non-existent, except some small tumours could be seen again in my lungs, which I found a bit worrying but they were in all likelihood inflammation, so my oncologist said they were nothing to worry about. I had been suffering with diarrhoea again and also with the raised blood pressure, my oncologist, and also my family who were at the consultation, decided that I should drop the Votrient to 400mg (2 tablets) a day to give the body a bit of a rest. So we did that and it certainly helped get everything under control again. The thing with targeted drugs is that you can play around with them and drop the dosage for a bit, or stop them altogether and then restart them again, or up the dosage if you see more activity or disease progression.

At this time due to the diarrhoea I had taken to wearing what I call my big girl pants. They are big, incontinence nappy type things that are really safe to keep any leakage at bay. Where we are now living, (which is easier to get to and from treatments and much easier to get to my office) in Tseung Kwan O in the New Territories. Fondly known as Junk Bay before, it is built on the reclaimed land from said bay. To get anywhere out of this area by car the quickest way to travel is through a tunnel. You can also use the MTR (Tube), but I tend to avoid it, as there are too many people coughing and spluttering at all times of the year, so it's too easy to catch germs. In the morning when everyone is going to work, the traffic in the tunnel is pretty bad and you can be stuck in a traffic queue for a quite a long time. So mentally, getting in a taxi and getting to work became, and still is quite challenging. I know that once we turn on to the tunnel road there is no way to get off it and so if I have to go to the loo, there is no way to get to a toilet and I have to hold it. This probably makes things worse, as even before I've left home I am worrying what the traffic will be like. I have only once been in a situation of desperation. Before we turn on to the tunnel road there is a roundabout and I had to get the taxi driver to turn around there and take me home, where I just made it back to the toilet. I now have a spare pair of clothes at work, including underwear, in case I do have a disaster, but my big girl pants are now my best friend. It's more a confidence issue, I think now, or a comfort blanket, but I always wear them whenever I am going out to somewhere that I know it will not be easy to rush to a toilet. On bad days I need to wear them all day at home in case I can't even make it to the toilet on time. I have to chuckle some days when I am in the office sitting in a serious meeting, or at one time doing a serious presentation and thinking, 'If they only knew what I had under my dress!' But I think that's what we hide sometimes and it is what people don't see. On the outside you look fine and they don't really understand how damaged you are underneath your strong and healthy looking exterior. It is also very hard mentally with diarrhoea, as you are chained to the nearest toilet and constantly worrying about this. There are medications but sometimes they don't always work.

Life continued as normal as possible and I had my next PET/CT scan to see what was going on. Unfortunately, because we had dropped the dosage of the Votrient, the lymph node in the porta hepatis had shot up in activity again to 9.63, which was bad news. Although dropping the Votrient had helped with my diarrhoea it hadn't helped with the cancer. However, all other tumours had gone, but we still had inflammation in the lungs, which was frustrating.

The question now was what could we do with this damn lymph node to sort it out. My oncologist said that there was new research showing that if targeted stereotactic body radiotherapy (SBRT) was used this would kick start the immune system again and get the T-Cells to wake up and attack the tumour, plus also causing what is called an apscopic effect where this would also attack any other underlying microscopic tumours in the body. The thought of using radiotherapy again, in my mind was a no, no, as I'd felt so unwell on my last treatment and also it had been totally ineffective. If anything, because it had lowered my immune system so much, it had caused the tumours in my liver to grow so fast. Also because the tumour had the KRAS mutation and research shows that because this mutation repairs its DNA so fast, it is immune to radiotherapy treatment I was really against it. However, after discussing with my cousin in UK, who is also an oncologist working with immunotherapy drugs and she explained how it would work in detail and that she had patients with the KRAS mutation who were on immunotherapy, where this kind of treatment had worked I decided since it wouldn't make things worse, I would give it a go.

I discussed with my surgeon whether he could take it out and he said he had done this kind of operation on a patient before, but she had no other active disease and had been cured. Now that I was stage 4 and it would also mean coming off my cancer drugs, he didn't think it was a feasible option. Neither did my oncologist. My surgeon also said that he could open me up and find that the node was fused to the portal hepatic artery and would not be able to take it out anyway, so a lot of discomfort and hassle for nothing. So that idea was 'parked' for now.....

My oncologist referred me to a nice young radiology doctor whom I met with to discuss the SBRT treatment and we arranged all the costs with the insurance company and got a Guarantee of Payment letter provided to the Hong Kong Sanatorium. I was returning there for treatment, since this is the best hospital in Hong Kong for radiotherapy treatment. They have also now been building a Proton Therapy Centre off site which will be excellent.

I did have to chase up the hospital accounts as they had a problem with the wording in the GOP, so once again always have to be on the ball with all these private hospitals accounts departments.

I first needed to go in to be measured up and to also have a test for the Assisted Breathing Control machine (ABC) so they could set it up. Basically because the SBRT is a very intensive and targeted radiotherapy, the less area it has to target for important organs the better. This meant that I was required to hold my breath intermittently throughout treatment. My oncologist and the radiology doctor said 'Don't worry, it's just like you were diving.' You have a peg on your nose and you breathe through a tube, and then occasionally have to hold your breath while the radiotherapy machine is working.

This process entailed me lying on a bed with a CT machine. First they scrunched a kind of airbag around me, which became my body bag which was used each time I had treatment to line me up. I also had the obligatory black lines drawn on my body again to direct where the machine should be placed. I needed to hold my breath so that the machine could measure this and know when to cut off the air in the real treatment. You can't breathe in too deeply or too shallow; it has to be just right. I was required to take 10 breaths and hold for 20 seconds. With my already inflamed and compromised lungs it was very difficult, I felt as if I was suffocating. The team handling this kept saying 'Keep going you can do this,' and I kept saying 'No I really can't'. To the point where I ended up in tears because they obviously weren't listening to me. It was horrible. I asked the radiotherapy doctor if I could drop the breath-holding down to 15 seconds and he agreed that it could be adjusted.

I even practised this at home but still found 15 seconds a struggle.

The treatment was planned for 5 sessions, one day on and one day off. I did tell my boss that I would work from home on the off day, but was so exhausted that it didn't happen.

When we came to the actual treatment I was called in after changing into a gown, laid down on the radiotherapy table in my mould so that the alignment was right, and my body jiggled around a bit to get the black lines on my body correct and then had the peg clipped on my nose and the breathing tube inserted.

Because we dropped the breath holding down to 15 seconds, I had to do in total 35 breath holdings per treatment. The radiologist tells you to hold your breath, then you breathe in and the machine starts and zaps the relevant area and then he tells you to release your breath. Each treatment entailed 3 rounds of 10 breaths and then one of 5 to start with, to align the machine.

After every treatment I would feel exhausted and invariably leave with a headache. If anyone tries that themselves you will find that you become lightheaded and headachy if you have to constantly breath in and hold your breath.

When I got up off the table after each treatment I could feel that radiated area burning, which is apparently normal. That week had to have been the toughest I have had to endure yet and I wouldn't do that again. SBRT, yes, but not using an ABC Machine. Never, ever, ever again. I said to my friends that it was worse than having half my liver removed and that is the truth, honestly. It was ghastly, for me anyway.

You do get to control the machine, which is one good thing, as when you are asked to take a breath you push the button on a hand-held device you are given, which gives the machine the go ahead to radiate. Then you are told to let go of the breath and the button on the hand-held device which stops the machine. So had I thought I couldn't hold my breath, or needed to take the breathing device out of my mouth, I could at least have some comfort in knowing that the radiotherapy machine would stop and I wouldn't be breathing at the wrong time and it zapping something that it shouldn't.

What probably made it worse was the fact that my radiology doctor told me that I could get diarrhoea or nausea while on this treatment, as the radiotherapy was hitting close to the stomach and upper intestine. Having this tube in the mouth and taking these breaths while feeling continuously nauseous was awful.

In general many ladies from my cancer support group have said that radiotherapy is much worse than chemotherapy treatment and I would absolutely agree with that. But this is of course is not the case for everyone.

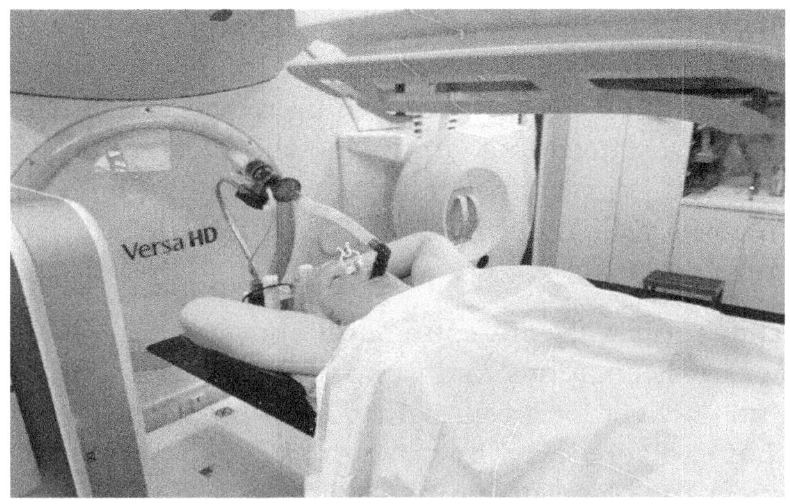

Me having the SBRT with the Assisted Breathing Control Machine

While I was visiting the hospital at that time, due to my exhaustion (which is a side effect of the immunotherapy), my oncologist suggested that I do a sleep study, as she suspected I might have sleep apnea. I found I wasn't sleeping well and at night would suddenly wake up and found I was taking a big breath out, which had jerked me awake. Having put on a lot of weight, as mentioned before, I don't think this helped at all.

The sleep test was really fascinating as you are put into a private sleep test room with a camera filming all night. You are rigged up to loads of sensors, which are stuck on your head, eyelids, jaw, heart area, legs and wearing an oximeter on the finger for the pulse. All these little sensors then read what your brain is doing when you sleep. If your eyelids flicker, if your jaw grinds or moves, what your heart is doing plus pulse and oxygen level and lots of other things. The only one thing which was fun is that if you need to go to the loo you have to have a bed pan, as you are all wired up, so quite difficult to cover your modesty while being filmed, but had to be done!

The result was interesting and showed that I have severe sleep apnea and wake up 57 times a minute and only get for a full night 60% of proper sleep, so that explained why I was so tired. Sleep apnea can affect the blood pressure (raising it) and the heart. I have since been told by a sleep specialist in the UK that if I lose weight this could be curative, but this is tricky at the moment due to the drug weight gain.

I was recommended to try a CPAP machine, which I am hiring on a monthly basis at the moment to test it out. I have to put a mask over my nasal area and breathe through my nose. The machine is continually pumping air through (I also have a humidifier attached to mine so the air is not too dry) and then when my airway becomes compressed, which is what causes me to wake up, the machine increases the air pressure to open the airway up. I know many people who use this to great affect, so I am just getting used to it at the moment. Celki air, who I rent it from say if I can do 4 hours with it on at the moment, then that is good to start with. The machine has a card reader so they can read it and see what happens at night when I am breathing. The machine and accessories are very compact and will be easy to take with me when travelling.

Life went on as normal except about a month later I had absolutely awful pains in my diaphragm area, like a really bad indigestion which just wouldn't go. I contacted my radiotherapy doctor and he told me to go to the nearest private hospital, which was St Teresa's and he would meet me there. We did an ECG and it did look like the heart was bumping about a bit, but he said nothing to worry about, so I was given some medicine and sent home. By the next morning it was still very painful. My oncologist contacted me, as she had heard about the night before and asked for my ECG. Once she saw it she said, 'Ooh, you'd better come into the clinic as you could be having a mini heart attack'. I immediately got in a taxi and went to see her. I had another ECG and blood tests, which can give an indication on the risk of heart attack, but all seemed normal, thank goodness. She gave me some stronger medication a proton pump inhibitor, which I wasn't supposed to take with my targeted drug, but we stopped that drug to sort out this pain. As mentioned, it seems that it is very normal practice to stop and start targeted drugs. Hence the name, so that on occasions when you need a rest from them for whatever reason they can be stopped for a while.

At this time I was invited to go and speak at a press conference for the launch of a new ovarian cancer drug, a PARP Inhibitor called Zejula. PARP inhibitors are historically used for patients with the BRCA1 or BRCA2 gene, which is usually hereditary from either mother or father. If you have the BRCA gene you are at risk of getting cancer in the ovaries and the breasts, but there is only a smaller percentage of women that have this genetic mutation, approximately 5-10% of breast cancer patients and 15% of ovarian cancer patients. However, Zejula has clinical evidence showing that it can also be effective on women without the BRCA mutation. My oncologist still said that you would have more success if you had other BRCA-like mutations which I don't, so it wasn't a drug that we could consider. Having also read up on the side effects, because I have been so heavily pre-treated with chemotherapy, it could also cause some pretty hard core life threatening side effects, so I think not a drug for me. In Hong Kong, it is pretty taboo, to talk about cancer, people just don't like to be open about it. But for me that is not the case, I believe that the more open people are about it, the more help and support they can get and also more help they can give other cancer patients. I do quite often get approached to speak or give my patient story to the Press.

Unfortunately, the day I was supposed to be at the Press conference the whole episode with the heart happened and I was at my oncologists having my ECG etc. I felt terrible for letting the PR agency down, but this is the challenge with cancer, you never really know what the next day will bring. For me being a high performer in both life and work I find it very hard to lose control of my body and not to be able to plan. I am getting better but just hate letting people down. The PR and drug company, of course, understood and the MC still read out my story, which was good. I put myself through this because I really want to be the patient voice and am determined to raise awareness from the patient point of view for ovarian cancer whenever I can.

I also in May that year accompanied my oncologist and Tracy to a Press conference to raise awareness of NG Sequencing. I know I have said this already, but for anyone who is diagnosed your first step must be to get a biopsy done and send your tumour samples to Foundation Medicine to get your genomic mutations tested. Without this information, how can your oncologist have the best chance to treat you, if they don't know what's driving the tumour proliferation. If you don't have a tumour sample a liquid biopsy can be taken and that sent off. These are done for blood cancers too, when you have no tumour tissue to send.

The Press were all Asian so I never saw the write ups, although my local colleagues at work kept coming up to me saying 'I read about you in the newspaper!' So, I hope it did raise awareness of the NG Sequencing test locally and encouraged patients to use it.

I was approached though by a lot of ladies originally from Mainland China, who are now living in other places such as Europe or USA, who read the article and I am very pleased that I can support them. I hope eventually we are able to translate this book into Chinese.

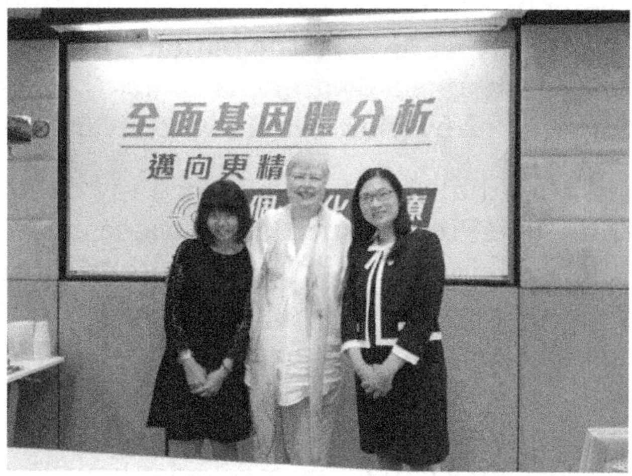

Me, Tracy and my oncologist at the Foundation Medicine press conference

In Hong Kong for Breast Cancer Awareness Month in October, there is loads of publicity and fund raising but I have never seen any publicity regarding global Ovarian Cancer Awareness Day which is the 8th May. Only one day, but nothing, so it is my goal to change this!

Back to the journey! Life carried on, although I could feel that my body was getting more inflamed by the immunotherapy drug. More frequent diarrhoea and a very unsettled stomach, with frequent gastric reflux and indigestion, with a feeling that I constantly had something stuck in my throat, harder to breathe with inflamed lungs, feeling my teeth 'jangling' all the time, so this wasn't very pleasant.

When we had my next PET scan (we didn't bother with a CT scan since my cancer was so stable) the results were really good. It seemed that the SBRT had worked, thankfully! All the SBRT hassle was worth it! And the porta hepatis lymph node had reduced in activity to 2.93. However, the size remained the same. I also still had the inflammation in my lungs and from my oesophagus right down to my lower bowel you could see every twist and turn. It was hugely inflamed. Tracy commented that she'd not seen a bowel so inflamed like that before, not even with bowel cancer patients! So this explained the constant diarrhoea and the reflux.

My drug Keytruda is usually administered for 2 years as mentioned before and then stopped. Then if progression starts again it is administered again. I was off by 3 treatments so my oncologist said she would proceed with these and then we would stop, or really space out the treatment for a while. Also, it was difficult to say what was really happening with the porta hepatis lymph node, due to all the inflammation in the body. The 2.93 reading could actually now be inflammation, so my oncologist was going more on the size. If it gets down to 2cms then this can be considered normal. She thinks that the SBRT could still be bubbling around, so the lymph node may still get smaller and more inactive. The good thing is that it has always been contained even when at an activity level of 21, so that is all that matters really. I had hoped for NED (No Evidence of Disease) status or remission, but stable is also good enough. Patients live for many years with stable disease so let's not get greedy as stable is good.

For me the news was really excellent and I could start thinking about a longer-term future and make more plans which had been difficult before. My oncologist also gave me a special dispensation to fly! So this year the whole family are flying back to UK for the Christmas holiday, which will be lovely as I haven't seen many of my friends and family from the UK for almost 7 years, only the ones who have visited us here in Hong Kong. A big event to look forward to for sure!

Unfortunately, though, on my next Keytruda treatment everything suddenly seemed to tip over the top. I was really ill for about 2 weeks. So fatigued I couldn't get out of bed, vomiting, diarrhoea, reflux and indigestion. The reflux was so bad I actually burnt the back of my throat, so swallowing was really painful and I constantly felt like I had something stuck in my throat. I had toothache, joints aching, bladder sore and kept weeing because it was so irritated, which meant I also couldn't sleep at night as constantly up and down to the loo, headaches – everything. My blood pressure was raised from the Votrient and on 2 occasions I suddenly, out of nowhere, got a banging headache like my head would explode, was violently sick, the left side of my face went red and hot and I felt really dizzy. You would almost have thought I was having a stroke, but as I am on blood thinners that was highly unlikely.

I wasn't able to get into the office or even to see my oncologist as I didn't feel well enough and also with the diarrhoea so difficult to even leave the house. Although I felt unwell I also got cabin fever being stuck at home. I did at one point think to myself bring it on, if you want to kill me cancer, then get on with it. I don't want to live with this kind of quality of life. These thoughts were only fleeting and as always, I went to my mum, who was so supportive. Her take on it all is, 'Hey you have a chronic disease here, you are entitled to feel unwell. No one has to be happy and positive all the time or put a brave face on things, you are entitled to have a bad day, don't be so hard on yourself.' That is my advice to anyone else too. Allow yourself to be fed up sometimes and to have a bad day. We are after all human and not some super power that is invincible.

When I did finally get to see my oncologist, we did discuss treatment with steroids which is usual practice for inflammation, but due to previous steroid treatment, when I had my interim ultrasound checks we saw non-alcoholic fatty liver, which can be caused by steroids, so we preferred to leave it to try and heal by itself. There are other drugs that can be used for patients who cannot tolerate steroids but I was not offered these.

I did start a really strict anti-inflammatory diet, which seemed to help. Curcumin, the ingredient for Turmeric, is always recommended to bring down inflammation but as I have mentioned it also thins the blood so no good for me. Although my dear long standing friend Emilia, who has an organic business in Indonesia, did give me some fresh turmeric root when she visited recently, which I believe is much better to use than supplements, and not so strong, so we are using that in my anti -inflammatory recipes. The fabulous Dr Michael Mosely has written a book called 'The Clever Guts Diet' and his wife Dr Claire Bailey has written 'The Clever Guts Diet Recipe Book' so we do use that a lot to repair my gut. It has a lot of recipes with seaweed, fresh turmeric, fermented foods – all good for lowering inflammation. Our gut is the hub of our body, if that's out of kilter then so is everything else.

During this time of feeling ill, I took the Votrient on and off, but my blood pressure remained high.

I started to feel better, but then my heart, which had been jumping around and speeding up/slowing down occasionally, and had started to do this more right after the SBRT, suddenly seemed to go a bit strange too. It really got worse and became unmanageable. Both my legs swelled up, my feet and toes became quite painful as the skin stretched over them, so I put my compression stockings on to help. I booked an appointment with my cardiologist as thought it best to discuss with him. The day before my appointment I felt really good, no inflammation pain, lots of energy and thought 'Oh no this is typical! It's all calmed down now and he won't see anything!' However, when I lay down to do the ECG check, it went crazy! Speeded up and bumping around so it was all captured. On the ECG, it showed at one point that my pulse rate was 250!!!!

My cardiologist is a lovely, maturer man and very calm with a wealth of knowledge. He listened to all my symptoms and said that this could have been down to the chemotherapy, the targeted drug Votrient (this is a side effect) or even the SBRT. I could even have had an underlying problem, which the drugs and radiotherapy had perhaps exacerbated. It looked like my atrial fibrillation (arrhythmia) had got a lot worse. He was a bit concerned about the general condition of my heart so ordered a CT scan to check for coronary artery disease. He also gave me some stronger pills to help with the arrhythmia. They did work, but I also needed to up the dosage of my Concor to help.

I also went to see my oncologist who did another ECG and checked my bloods again. I don't mention my CA125 marker too much, as it can't always be relied upon, but this had remained under 5 after the SBRT. In fact, the lowest it got to was 2.1 so we were really doing good in terms of the cancer, it was more the side effects which were the worry.

My oncologist advised that the 2 drugs I was on were on a Phase 1 drug trial, I hadn't even looked this up as I trusted her completely so didn't know this, but she told me the trial had been stopped because of the toxicity of the drugs! So, I had done really well to survive on the combination for 2 years without any major adverse side effects.

As I end this part of the journey for now, we are leaving it that I need to go and talk to my cardiologist about next steps to remedy my heart problem. I am now off all cancer drugs and have been for about 2 months. I was due to stop or really space out the Keytruda anyway. My cancer status is all stable and no new disease for over a year, just the porta hepatis lymph node is the one to watch. Yes, I do have a big fear that I will have tumours springing back up now that we are on no drugs and I do accept that this will happen, unfortunately, as I am stage 4 but at the moment we just have to watch and wait. As an interim between scans we can do an ultrasound, particularly on my liver, as I always worry about tumours there as they are fast growing due to the blood supply, but they also regress pretty quickly once on a drug regime too.

I guess the hope is that the T-Cells are now re-programmed to go and seek out the tumours which cannot hide behind a protein barrier and kill them, but from past experience we also need to add in a catalyst to help.

I have written to the oncologist in the UK to see if she has any ideas on which drugs we might use going forward, as she is the expert on ovarian cancer and runs a lot of drug trials herself in the UK.

Looking at it logically it is step by step for now......

Get the heart sorted out and then review whether we still administer a top up for the immunotherapy, and also which other catalyst drug we can use. There are so many drug trials happening out there, so I hope we do have another drug to move on to and in the meantime the cancer stays stable with no little surprises. The body is powerful and so is the immune system. It has great healing properties and at the moment it is just saying to me, 'Hey, it's all too much I need a break from all these drugs, I've been battered for 5 years I need a rest', so that's what it will have.

It is getting harder to get up every day and go to work as the fatigue is incredible. I am hugely forgetful, find it hard to concentrate and process conversations, have lost my confidence a bit but I am determined to keep going and try to lead as normal a life as possible.

So, I guess it is watch this space for now.......

I recently read something from a cancer patient which I think is very relevant.

Imagine that one day someone comes up behind you and puts a gun at the back of your neck. They say that they are now going to hold that gun there for the rest of your life. For most of the time you will forget it is there, except for that slight touch of metal. However, sometimes they will just remind you that they are there, they say, by increasing the pressure on your neck or even cocking the trigger if they really want to scare you, but it will always be there at the back of your neck.

This is oh, so true. Even if you go into remission or are cured that gun will always be there reminding you, just niggling away at the back of your mind.

But that shouldn't stop you living and enjoying your life to the full, as who knows how long we have all got; live in the moment!

I was given a card previously with the quote: 'LIFE'S NOT ABOUT WAITING FOR THE STORM TO PASS, IT'S ABOUT LEARNING HOW TO DANCE IN THE RAIN'.

Dance and laugh every day readers that's what our time on this earth is really about!..............................

Chapter Six

The Continuing Journey

Since finishing the full text of the First Edition at page 120, I have been blessed to have almost sold out of the 300 copies I printed initially. Therefore, I have the luxury of correcting some typos! And to give a full update of where we are now in the journey in this Second Edition, as we reprint.

My cardiologist investigated the heart and it is in very good condition, so no risk of heart attack. In fact I have zero calcification in my arteries, which is way above average for a female of my age. It's an electrical problem, which is more a risk of a stroke. We tried several heart drugs, but settled on a higher dose of Concor, which seemed to work (and it doesn't interact with my cancer drugs) to control it, plus I am now injecting Clexane 2 times a day into my leg, to ensure that we have no more blood clots. I have taken diuretics for the foot and leg swelling which has worked, so they are now back to normal. We had an ultrasound of my liver and abdomen and saw no new visible tumours or fluid build-up (ascites) in the abdomen. We also did a CT of the lungs which looked OK, still showing a bit of inflammation. More importantly the porta hepatis lymph node was still the same size, as it was on the PET scan in February. I am very relieved that we have had no visible progression for the time I have been off the drugs!

The cancer marker had risen slightly from 2.1 to 4.2 and then to 5.2, so we tried 400mg daily of Votrient to see what happened. Unfortunately, 2 days after taking it, my heart speeded up and this lasted for the longest it has so far (5 minutes), at 148 beats a minute and I felt like I was going to pass out. I was in the office so was panicking what to do. Call an ambulance or just wait until it settled. But it did calm down after the 5 minutes and then we were back to normal rhythm. I booked in to see my cardiologist right away and rushed off to see him. I also called my brother who said 'Just stop the tablets again and see if you have any reaction'. I also WhatsApped my oncologist to let her know. When I saw the cardiologist he said the same thing 'Stop the drug and see what happens'. After stopping it, all was fine again, so back to the drawing board. Unfortunately, Votrient and another drug Avastin are anti angiogenic so perfect for ovarian cancer, but also affect the heart. There are other Tyrosine Kinase Inhibitors like Lenvitinib and Axitinib that are also good, but they all cause arrhythmia, so with the current state of my heart not good really. A solution is to do a small surgery called RFA, similar to what I had on my liver, but this time I guess you could almost call it 'soldering' some veins in the heart. This creates scar tissue to block the abnormal electrical signals, to get it to beat normally again. My cardiologist said that the risk was too great for the potential benefit, as it doesn't always work.

Since we were at an impasse with the drugs i.e. Anything except the Keytruda would affect my heart, we still needed to look at fixing this. I did feel we were on the magic roundabout a bit and I expected Florence or Zebedee to pop up at any moment. 'Stop the merry go round I want to get off please!'. I decided to take matters into my own hands and booked an appointment with a younger cardiologist at The Adventist hospital, where they have a specialist arrhythmia centre, for a second opinion. He was director of this department. He said that RFA would be a good option with an 80-85% chance of success, so good enough odds for me!

This procedure can be done awake under local anaesthetic or asleep under general anaesthetic. My cardiologist opted for a general. The plan was to stop the atrial fibrillation (the speeding up and the dangerous one) and also a 'flutter' when my heart skipped a beat, which was more minor at that time.

In I went to The Adventist again, with GOP in place and the luxury of a private room. I went down for the surgery at around 2pm, and then woke up in the operating theatre feeling very cold. Was wheeled back up to my room and noticed on the clock that it said 10pm! I couldn't quite believe it! I was very stressed as had said I would call my mum, as she would be so worried, if she hadn't heard anything. In the end, she called the hospital to find out how I was. She was told that they didn't have anyone of that name on the ward, to which my mum said

‘Erm she checked in with you this morning! So you must have her somewhere!’ Apparently, I had disappeared into some black hole it seemed! And then I was being wheeled up and they were able to tell her that I had just come out of theatre, and that all was well. The lovely Scottish nurse wasn’t working unfortunately, as I know she would have been able to advise mum as to what was happening.

When I got up to my room I was just shivering and shivering which was horrible. Apparently, this was the side effects of the anaesthetic, but it was very unpleasant as I’d never experienced this before with any other GA. I was then left to rest and hooked up to an ECG machine, which was monitored in the ICU unit, just in case of any issues.

I woke up suddenly in the night with all the nurses rushing in and could feel my heart beating really weirdly and fast. All I could think of was ‘Oh no! we’ve made it worse’ and feeling pretty scared. The nurses were great and said it’s OK, we are on the phone to the cardiologist to get advice on the drugs to give you. They administered them and then we were all back to normal. It was quite reassuring to be monitored in ICU though.

My cardiologist had kindly instructed the nurses to insert a catheter into my bladder, so I could sleep that night and rest.

In the morning the heart was still bobbing around, but he told me not to worry it was just really inflamed and it would calm down. It did after a week actually so he was right. The bruising on my leg was unbelievable! Right down the thigh, looked like I'd been in a car crash! That was just from having a small catheter inserted into my groin. My Arnica did wonders though and the bruising soon went a greeny yellow and then disappeared.

Also, he had taken longer than he thought, as it was difficult to find the 'flutter' and as I have found out it, is more effective and better to do this with the patient awake. More to follow on that shortly!

I stayed for 2 days in hospital and then home. The cardiologist went over the GOP value due to the extra time in the operating theatre, however the joy of being at The Adventist, meant that they could phone up the insurance company and get all the money sorted out. Having been told I could be discharged at 11am, I did in fact have to wait until 3pm to be discharged, as we were waiting on the insurance company to approve the extra money.

I have now built a good relationship with the insurance company's team in Hong Kong, so did e-mail them to hurry them up also.

Once home, I was put on an antiarrhythmic drug called Cordarone to help with getting the heart to beat normally again, plus antibiotics to help curb any infection. It did bounce around for quite a while until it settled and then all seemed well.

I heard back from the oncologist in the UK and she said that new research is showing that the ARID1A 'loss', is now definitely proving to be the main driver for clear cell ovarian cancer. She is doing a trial in the UK, called The Patriot Trial which is proving successful. It is at late phase 1/early phase 2 trial stage and using an ATR inhibitor. In Asia, apparently, there are 2 doctors in Singapore researching into this and so she has recommended that I contact them for more information. This is an exciting new development, and as clear cell OC is more prevalent in Asian women, it is good to see oncologists doing more research and trials here in Asia. My oncologist when she worked in the public hospital system ran loads of drug trials, so when I mentioned regarding the ATR inhibitor, I could see a dreamy look come over her face and the cogs in the brain were turning!

We then decided to do another scan to see the state of play and then see how we could proceed with the drugs.

To our amazement, the porta hepatis lymph node had reduced further in size to 1cm, and also in activity! When I met with my oncologist regarding this with my brother, she said it was great news! However, I still needed to keep on the Keytruda despite it still inflaming my body and making me ill, since the porta hepatis lymph node was still there. When we left the consultation, I said to my brother 'So does that mean I am NED?' to which he replied, 'Well I guess so!' my oncologist seemed very cautious about it which was odd, as previously she had said if the size got down to less than 2cm then she would judge that it was inactive. I assume that oncologists are just being cautious as a matter of principal. I so wanted that damn lymph node to disappear altogether! I visualised it just fading away and kept that image and goal in my mind.

I set up a call with one of the doctors in Singapore, but as the porta hepatis lymph node was no longer active, we didn't really need to consider more drugs at this time apart from the Keytruda.

He was such a nice guy and so knowledgeable about clear cell ovarian cancer. A definite oncologist to add to my arsenal of experts. My plan is to go to Singapore in the summer and see him in person. I lived there for a year and loved it and have promised to take my mum to Gardens By The Bay, as a Bristol based company designed it and before she came out to Hong Kong, she went to a talk to hear how they went about it all. Since then she has always wanted to visit.

Several points he touched on were interesting. Only 30% of his patients had responded to Keytruda as a single agent. Patients with the ARID1A 'loss' and PIK3CA genomic mutation (like I have) responded well. Also in the lab, he noticed that there were a subset of cells in clear cell ovarian cancer, which were angiogenic or immunogenic and that the patients with the angiogenic subset, responded very well to the immunotherapy. He also said that he had run a trial in Singapore with an ATR Inhibitor on patients with ARID1A loss and none of them had responded! So that was enough for me to take that particular drug off the list! I do have a friend with clear cell ovarian cancer who is on the Patriot Trial, is Stage 3C and has been stable for 2 years. However, she is still unclear as to whether she has the ARID1A loss (they don't seem to be so open in the UK to giving out information), and the trial was for patients with solid tumours from a range of cancers, so she may be the only one with clear cell that has had success. It's not enough evidence for me to try it, especially with the doctor in Singapore's input. He did query why I was still having top ups of the Keytruda, as the cut off is supposed to be 2 years, but I said it was for maintenance. He did agree that he saw no harm in continuing with it, if I could cope with the side effects. If my cancer recurred again, he suggested I add in Avastin however, I know my oncologist was concerned about me having a brain bleed with this drug as more risk.

I think I mentioned previously about the doctor in the USA who has already moved on from the immunotherapy drugs Opdivo and Keytruda and is looking into other drugs such as OX40 Agonist and injecting directly into the tumour together with a TLR (Toll Like Receptor). Without repeating what he has in his book, for anyone interested in the immunotherapy route, I would strongly recommend that you read it. 'The Immunotherapy

Revolution', The Best New Hope for Saving Cancer Patients Lives – by Dr Jason Williams. If I have a recurrence then I will seriously look into having treatment with him, providing I have accessible tumours. You only need a one-time injection into the tumour and then off you go. He also adds in Cryoablation, or SBRT is just as good, to give a 'kick start'. He was only doing these treatments in New Mexico as not allowed to do them in the USA, but he is now doing them in Thailand, so much nearer and more realistic travel wise for me.

He also has some good tips on supplements to enhance the effectiveness of immunotherapy. It's primarily about getting a healthy gut biome and eating lots of fibre. I now take FOS prebiotic in the evening, have reduced my probiotics to only 2-3 weekly and they need to include Bifidobacterium longum and breve, added in a cranberry supplement, he suggests omega 3 but I always have salmon for breakfast so that's covered, a handful of cashews a day which contain anacardic acid and pancreatic enzymes. However, the pancreatic enzymes made me feel nauseous so stopped them. There is a limit to what I will take if it makes me feel unwell.

So, I feel relaxed about my armoury going forward.

Unfortunately, after about 3 months of having the RFA to my heart, no more speeding up but I had the jumping and flutter again, and it was quite severe, i.e. 3,000 jumps overnight that we monitored on the holter.

My cardiologist said this wasn't really safe and he had struggled to find the flutter under GA, so suggested we did more RFA but with me awake this time. Not a pleasant thought but the flutter wasn't manageable. Also with heart problems I would be discounted from any drug trials, so I agreed that we do another RFA.

I was so terrified the day I went in for this. He said he would start in the evening as this is when the flutter was at its worst, so I went down at 4pm to theatre. In The Adventist hospital again and a private room for comfort.

The main thing I have to say is that it is incredibly, incredibly boring! My friend's husband has had it done and said he could see the screen with all the heart mapping being done, but because I said I felt a bit dizzy and drunk when the strong local anaesthetic was administered, I then had 2 big X-Ray units blocking my vision!

Once on the operating table you are given local anaesthetic in your right groin and then the catheter is inserted. You can't feel anything except the cardiologist pushing down hard on your groin. From time to time through the procedure it would ache, so I would say can I have some more local anaesthesia please. Once the catheter gets to the heart you have a funny sensation like your heart is jumping, but it is just the catheter mapping your heart. Then your heart is really speeded up, uncomfortably so, to make it flutter. Once the cardiology team see something, the cardiologist runs round and says, 'Does that feel like a jump?' and you say 'Yes' and off he trots to view where the break is in the electrical connection. After that there was an awful lot of talking in Cantonese! The anaesthesist them gave me some 'juice', which made me feel drunk and then I heard my cardiologist say 'ablate.' You don't feel anything in the heart, but it gave me toothache and also nerves in my shoulder were jangling a bit, but otherwise no problem. This went on for hours! Until at midnight! We were done and I was wheeled back up to my room. This time we had tagaderm wrapped tightly around my leg and it did work as I had no bruising. However, we had stopped my Clexane injections a day earlier also, which I think helped. I was once again rigged up with an ECG connected to ICU and monitored. Again, the heart started bumping, but we knew from the previous RFA, that this would happen.

This time I called in advance down to accounts to check the GOP and they advised that 'Yes' the cardiologist had gone over the amount again! But between myself and the accounts team, we managed to get approval from the insurance company quickly, and I was out the next day. Once again, I was on Cordarone and we have done holter checks monthly, everything did seem to be good.

I unfortunately caught really bad bronchitis from a colleague at work in November, (I wish these sick people would stay at home!), which got so bad I had to have a nebulizer to help me breathe. That set back any Keytruda treatments for a while!

Since myself and my family were going home to UK for Christmas, the first time in 7 years as not on Pazopanib anymore, my oncologist and I decided to do another PET/CT scan to check on status. I as always had scanxiety and I guess always will have, but just still being on only Keytruda concerned me.

When we got the results, my wish had come true and the portas hepatis lymph node was completely gone! I can now truly say that I am NVED, or as I like to call it 'No Visible Evidence of Disease!' My oncologist still wanted to keep up the Keytruda so I had only a 100mg before we flew, so I wouldn't have any bad side effects while in UK.

The other slight problem on my list to fix was the incisional hernia which is apparently very common when you've had abdominal surgery, as the abdomen wall gets weakened. It started quite small around 2017 and then wasn't a priority as bigger things to worry about, and also I was on Pazopanib, which needs to be stopped for about a month if you have surgery, so just wasn't top of the list. However, it did rip across the abdomen wall and got quite big and sore and it also prevented me from exercising and caused constipation. So I decided it needed fixing. We have just done this. The surgeon said he might have to do a bowel resection and it all sounded very major and painful. But actually, the surgery only took 2 and a half hours and was remarkably simple so he said. So that was all good. No pain really and able to move fairly freely after about 4 days. A bit tired after another general anaesthetic but otherwise very painless. I have decided to treat myself to a personal trainer this year, since I am now in remission, it is time to heal the body, lose weight and get my fitness level back.

The heart has been jumping around a bit again but this may be due to the general anaesthetic and the antibiotics so hopefully it will settle.

The book sales have been tremendous and I have raised a good amount of money for my two ovarian cancer charities, Target Ovarian Cancer in the UK and the Ovarian Cancer Research Alliance (OCRA) in USA, who both do a great deal of research into this silent killer. This is what we need, a way of detecting this disease earlier, so many women can be cured rather than symptoms arising at stage 4, when it is too late.

I have done a few book signings which went really well and am now selling the book in Bookazine a Hong Kong based book store. We also now have a website run by two of my lovely supporters, who have some other online businesses. I was waiting to complete this Second Edition and now that I have, will be looking at doing an eBook format and translating the book into Chinese.

My Top 10 Tips (which I should listen to more myself!):

1) Choose your oncologist well, it must be someone you can trust and work with.

2) Once you find a good one and choose a treatment regime, get your head down and stick with it, don't go seeking numerous second, third, fourth opinions as you will only confuse yourself as to which path to take. Although a second opinion is good to have.

3) Do your research – question, question and more questions!

4) Don't beat yourself up if you can't make appointments/let people down last minute. You have a chronic disease after all and people should understand this (particularly yourself!). It took me a long time to accept this.

5) Only spend time with people who make you feel good, you don't need to be with people who want to load their life problems on to you - just push back. It again took me a long time to learn to do this!

6) Be open about your disease and talk about it, it is not something you caused and you are not an outcast just because of it.

7) Have a good support system around you of fellow cancer patients as they truly know what you are going through.

8) Don't feel guilty when you eat the odd chocolate or cake – we do after all deserve a treat now and again.

9) Keep a private closed Facebook page or a journal of your journey, sometimes it helps to write it all down and get it out of the system.

10) Be prepared for lasting side effects – for me I am left with no short-term memory (I have to write everything down), find it hard to concentrate some days, it takes much longer to digest what people are saying to me and process the information, feel my brain is in a fog most days, arrhythmia, less strength in my grip and still peripheral neuropathy in my fingers, painful joints, osteopenia, risk of blood clots, a very sensitive bowel and a hernia on my right side on the incision across my belly from my second abdomen surgery (very common and is not caused by weight gain, that part of the abdomen is just weakened by surgery), it has now been fixed. But I am still ALIVE and that's all that matters!

Appendices:

Cancer Journey in Chronological Order:

Keyhole surgery performed in April 2014 and FIGO Stage 1 (Grade 2) endometroid of the ovary with clear cell component diagnosed.

Underwent optimal surgical debulking in Hong Kong ~ bilateral salpingo ~ oophorectomy, omentectomy and pelvic lymph nodes (0/10).

Received 6 cycles adjuvant chemotherapy (Carboplatin x 6, Paclitaxel x 4 ~ stopped due to peripheral neuropathy and DVT in left leg) completed October 2014.

PET-CT February 2015 showed mild uptake in a right peritoneal nodule.

May 2015, 2 x PET avid nodules ~ received 6 cycles of Gemcitabine/Capecitabine October 2015. Reduced activity noted after 2 cycles but disease progression on completion of 6 cycles in October 2015. July 2015 suffered DVT in right leg resulting in Pulmonary Embolism.

Underwent surgical debulking in Hong Kong 30th November 2015. 1/8 left obturator lymph nodes involved with clear cell carcinoma, 0/31 right pelvic lymph nodes and 0/8 left pelvic lymph nodes. Peritoneal sections showed no malignancy. Omental deposits showed haemorrhagic change only. 2014 histology confirms oestrogen receptor positive (6), progesterone receptor positive (8).

Completed secondary debulking surgery.

Adjuvant radiotherapy 18th January to 24th February 2016 by Varian True Beam, 6MV Photon, bilateral pelvic nodal regions, pre ~sacral nodal region, lower para ~aortic nodal region. Pre ~salvage surgery gross nodal region 50By, all other sites 45 By, 25 Fractions.

Surveillance PET~CT scan May 2016 shows liver metastases x 7 ranging from 1.38 cm to 10.3 cm in size.

Ultrasound guided core biopsy of the liver confirms metastatic clear cell carcinoma. PAX8 positive, focally positive for P53, WT1 negative, ER negative, PR negative.

June 2016 received 3 cycles Caelyx and Carboplatin. PET~CT scan staging August 2016 disease progression liver metastases x 8. Some uptake on smaller tumours with size reduction.

One cycle Pembrolizumab, 200mg, given August 2016.

September 8th left hemi hepatectomy and cholecystectomy performed plus right hepatectomy and RFA of 4 small tumour nodules in segment 6,7, 8 dome and caudate lobe. All tumours confined within liver capsule without breaching the serosa. No malignancy in gall bladder.

30th September 2016 follow up CT scan 1.79 cm suspected residual liver metastases detected.

10th October 2016 tumour in segment 5/8 ablated via subcostal approach with 15G STAR med electrode(3cm).

October to end December 2016 ~ 4 cycles Pembrolizumab, 200mg, 3 weekly (in total 5 received).

Surveillance PET ~CT scan 28th December 2016 showed disease progression – see PET/CT scan through immunotherapy.

6th January 2017 Abraxane weekly plus Pazopanib 2 tablets x 200mg daily, increasing to 3 tablets x 200mg daily. Abraxane stopped 4th May 2017 due to side effects.

11th May 2017 Pembrolizumab and Pazopanib 3 tablets x 200mg daily, Pembrolizumab 200mg every 3 weeks to date.

30th November 2018 - 5 cycles, one day on, one day off, Stereotactic Body Radiotherapy to porta hepatis lymph node due to increased activity.

March 2019 cancer drugs stopped due to heart problem. No progression found on lung CT scan and Liver/abdomen ultrasound.

May 2019 – Pembrolizumab and Pazopanib resumed at lower dosage but stopped again due to effect on heart.

June 2019 – one dose of Pembrolizumab administered as a top up.

17th June 2019 – RFA on heart.

July 2019 onwards - maintenance reduced dose of Pembrolizumab 150mg every 8 weeks indefinitely or until recurrence.

17th September 2019 – Second RFA on heart.

20th January 2020 – incisional hernia repair.

PET/CT Scans in chronological order once on Abraxane and Votrient combined for 4 months and then Votrient and Keytruda and then Keytruda alone. I think it is important to show these results and how on chemotherapy and a targeted drug I did have some partial metabolic response but it wasn't long term which has always been the case with the chemotherapy. Also with immunotherapy it is easy to get what looks like progression when it is in fact 'pseudo progression' caused by inflammation:

28th December 2016 – SUV Max references: Normal liver 4.27; Mediastinal blood pool 3.02

* SUV = Standardised update value; LD – Largest diameter; PD – Perpendicular diameter

Site	LD x PD (mm)	SUV Max	Remarks
R apical sub pleural nodule	4.7 x 4.1	2.22	
LUL sub aortic LN	10.0 x 9.1	3.86	
L sub aortic LN	15.3 x 9.9	4.13	
R interlobar LN	16.8 x 10.2 17.0 x 15.1	6.67 5.89	
L hilar LN	9.2 x 7.9	6.01	
L interlobar LN	8.0 x 5.6 12.2 x 10.7 15.2 x 8.2 11.7 x 11.2	4.15 6.45 7.09 6.58	
Precarinal LN	23.5 x 9.8	4.46	
Subcarinal LN	24.9 x 14.7	6.31	
L Subcarinal N	17.3 x 13.2	6.57	
Liver S8	18.3 x 15.4	11.01	S = Segment of liver
Liver S7	18.8 x 16.8	15.3	
Liver S6	24.4 x 24.3 19.8 x 19.6	21.9 8.53	
Liver S4/5	9.3 x 5.6	4.96	
Liver S4b	-	-	
Liver S3	-	-	
Liver S2	-	-	
Caudate lobe	-	-	
Porta-hepatis LN	27.5 x 13.7 21 x 16 12.7 x 12.3	10.37 15.1 8.59	
Anterior Abdominal wall	18.4 x 12.2	6.8	
Coeliac LN	10.4 x 8.5	6.12	
R mesenteric focus	8 x 7.6	6.40	
R ilium	-	4.47	right hip bone

13th March 2017 - SUV Max references: Normal liver 3.4; Mediastinal blood pool 2.21

Site	LD x PD (mm)	SUV Max	Remarks
R apical sub pleural nodule	3.4 x 2.7	No uptake	
LUL sub aortic LN	Resolved	No update	
L sub aortic LN	8.1 x 7.2	2.07	
R interlobar LN	16.8 x 10.2 17.0 x 15.1	6.67 5.89	
L hilar LN	14.9 x 10.9	3.99	
R hilar LN	10.3 x 10.2 15.5 x 10.4	4.27 4.36	new tumour – potentially inflammation
R interlobar	Present	-	
L interlobar LN	Present	-	
Precarinal LN	-	3.62	
Subcarinal LN	-	3.3	
L Subcarinal LN	12.5 x 9.7	4.42	
Liver S8	Resolved		S = Segment of liver
Liver S7	Resolved		
Liver S6	Resolved		
Liver S4/5	Resolved		
Liver S4b	Resolved		
Liver S3	Resolved		
Liver S2	Resolved		
Caudate lobe	Resolved		
Porta-hepatis LN	19 x 15.4	16.26	
Anterior Abdominal wall	20.3 x 14	5.84	
Coeliac LN	13.7 x 12.7	6.05	
R mesenteric focus	Resolved		
R ilium	Resolved		right hip bone

12th July 2017 - SUV Max references: Normal liver 3.87; Mediastinal blood pool 2.68

Taking Berberine which gave me diarrhea so Votrient not being absorbed

Site	LD x PD (mm)	SUV Max	Remarks
R apical sub pleural nodule	3.0	No uptake	
L hilar LN	-	3.57	
R hilar LN	-	3.72	potentially inflammation
Precarinal LN	- -	3.29 3.06	
Liver S8	10.9 x 10.7	15.58	S = Segment of liver
Liver S5	16.5 x 11.3	7.53	
Porta-hepatis LN	18.3 x 17.3	21.95	
Anterior Abdominal wall	14.6 x 13.9	7.93	
Retro Caval LN (Coeliac LN)	15.3 x 14.4	7.53	
L para aortic LN	18.4 x 15.4	9.62	new tumour potentially inflammation

22nd August 2017 - SUV Max references: Normal liver 4.29; Mediastinal blood pool 2.42

Came off Berberine, diarrhea resolved, follow up scan done close to July one to check difference.

Site	**LD x PD (mm)**	**SUV Max**	**Remarks**
R apical sub pleural nodule	-	No uptake	
R hilar LN (shotty)	- -	3.80 3.76	potentially inflammation
Precarinal LN (shotty)	- -	No uptake	
Subcarinal LN	-	No uptake	
Liver S8	10.9 x 10.6	8.43	S = Segment of liver
Liver S5	-	4.33 (delay) 4.95	
Porta-hepatis LN	17.5 x 13.7	16.42	
Anterior Abdominal wall	14.1 x 12.6	4.2	
Retro Caval LN (Coeliac LN)	13.5 x 10.2	5.76	
L para aortic LN	12.6 x 11.7	8.29	new tumour potentially inflammation

13th November 2017 - SUV Max references: Normal liver 4.13; Mediastinal blood pool 2.68

Site	LD x PD (mm)	SUV Max	Remarks
Liver S8	-	4.41 (4.33)	S = Segment of liver
Liver S5	-	4.79 (delay) 3.81	
Porta-hepatis LN	20.3 x 12.2	20.09	
Anterior Abdominal wall	11.6 x 9.7	3.17	
Retro Caval LN (Coeliac LN)	6.6 x 6.6	2.69	
L para aortic LN	9.9 x 8.7	2.86	potentially inflammation
Peritoneal deposit	11 x 9.8	4.51	new tumour potentially inflammation
R hilar LN (shotty)	-	2.44	potentially inflammation

2nd March 2018 - SUV Max references: Normal liver 4.27; Mediastinal blood pool 2.39

Site	LD x PD (mm)	SUV Max	Remarks
Liver S8	-	No abnormal uptake	S = Segment of liver
Liver S5	-	No abnormal uptake	
Porta-hepatis LN	13.1 x 10.0	8.67	
Anterior Abdominal wall	-	2.57	
Retro Caval LN (Coeliac LN)	-	2.64	
L para aortic LN	-	1.09	potentially inflammation
Peritoneal Deposit	Resolved	No abnormal update	potentially inflammation

18th July 2018 - SUV Max references: Normal liver 4.66; Mediastinal blood pool 3.05

Site	LD x PD (mm)	SUV Max	Remarks
Liver S8	-	No abnormal uptake	S = Segment of liver
Liver S5	-	No abnormal uptake	
Porta-hepatis LN	10.9 x 7.3	2.54	
Anterior Abdominal wall	-	1.98	
Retro Caval LN (Coeliac LN)	Resolved	No abnormal update	
L para aortic LN	Resolved	No abnormal update	potentially inflammation
RLL Sub pleural GGO	19.6	7.27	inflammation clear ground glass tumours
LLL GGO	-	4.01	inflammation clear ground glass tumours
R interlobar LN	12.4 x 8.8	4.22	inflammation
L interlobar LN	10.4 x 5.9	5.14	inflammation
Sub Carinal LN	10 x 6.5	4.32	inflammation

31st October 2018 - SUV Max references: Normal liver 4.87; Mediastinal blood pool 3.66

Site	LD x PD (mm)	SUV Max	Remarks
Porta-hepatis LN	15.5 x 8	9.63	
RLL atelectasis	-	4.08	inflammation
RML consolidation	-	2.49	inflammation
R interlobar LN/ L interlobar LN	Up to 12.9 x 11.1	6.14	inflammation
Sub Carinal LN	-	3.89	inflammation

22nd February 2019 - SUV Max references: Normal liver 4.47; Mediastinal blood pool 2.89

Site	LD x PD (mm)	SUV Max	Remarks
Porta-hepatis LN	15.0 x 8.8	2.93	
RLL atelectasis	-	2.62	inflammation
RML consolidation	-	2.70	inflammation
R interlobar LN/ L interlobar LN	9.2 x 8.8	4.01 3.85	inflammation
Sub Carinal LN	-	5.88	inflammation

10th July 2019 - SUV Max references: Normal liver 4.22; Mediastinal blood pool 2.94

Site	LD x PD (mm)	SUV Max	Remarks
Porta-hepatis LN	11.8 x 6.8	2.01	
RLL atelectasis	-	No uptake	inflammation
RML consolidation	-	No uptake	inflammation
R interlobar LN	14.4 x 13.8	2.33	inflammation
L interlobar LN	8.9 x 7.7	3.52	inflammation
Sub Carinal LN	10.4 x 7.5	2.02	inflammation

3rd December 2019 - SUV Max references: Normal liver 4.09; Mediastinal blood pool 3.27

Site	LD x PD (mm)	SUV Max	Remarks
Porta-hepatis LN	Resolved	Resolved	
RLL atelectasis	-	No uptake	
RML consolidation	-	No uptake	
R interlobar LN	15 x 13	2.89	inflammation
L interlobar LN	-	Resolved	
Sub Carinal LN	6	2.55	inflammation

NG Sequencing Test Results and Genomic Mutations:

First test done in August 2015 (funded by insurance company)

Genomic Mutations found:

PIK3CA; PTEN; ARID1A; MLL2; PIK3CG

Second test done in January 2018 (unfunded by the insurance company)

Additional genomic mutation found:

ERBB2 (HER2)

Tested in addition - Tumour Mutation Burden (TMB) which was Low, Microsatellite Status (MSI) which was Stable.

Third test done in April 2018 (unfunded by the insurance company)

Additional genomic mutation found:

KRAS

Separate test to the NG Sequencing, a test for PD1 receptivity which came out as 4% (low – i.e. PD1 negative) (all these statuses indicated that I was not a good candidate for PD1 immunotherapy treatment as a monotherapy). The PD1 test isn't always that reliable so can be used just as a guide.

Drugs:

Votrient (Pazopanib) – Protein Kinase Inhibitor. Works by interfering with pathways that signal certain cancer cells to grow. That way the cells in the body work and grow, is regulated by various enzymes called protein kinases.

Side effects I experienced – hypertension, diarrhoea, white hair, arrhythmia.

Keytruda (Pembrolizumab) – This drug works by targeting the protein on the surface of immune cells that stops them from attacking the malignant cells. The drug is an antibody which blocks the protein called PD-1 (programmed cell death) on the surface of the immune system T-cells. This prevents an activated PD-1 protein from stopping the immune response against the cancer.

Side effects I experienced: Incredible fatigue, diarrhea, weight gain, inflamed joints, flu like symptoms, continuous hot flushes.

Paclitaxol Chemotherapy – one of the taxane family which works by interference with the normal function of microtubules during cell division. It derives from the Pacific Yew tree.

Side effects I experienced: Severe peripheral neuropathy, memory loss, lack of concentration, fatigue, joint pain, total hair loss.

Carboplatin Chemotherapy – is from the family of drugs called antineoplastic which are platinum based and interfere with the duplication of DNA.

Side effects I experienced: Change in taste, fatigue.

Caelyx (doxorubicin) Chemotherapy – is part of the anthracycline and anti-tumour antibiotic family of drugs. It works in part by interfering with the function of DNA. It is often paired with another chemotherapy drug (in my case Carboplatin).

Side effects I experienced: We suspect damaged heart (arrhythmia).

Abraxane Chemotherapy – Is another drug from the taxane family and works in the same way as Paclitaxol but is a protein bound Paclitaxol.

Side effects I experienced: Peripheral neuropathy, hair thinning, fatigue.

Gemzar (Gemcitabine) Chemotherapy – is part of the nucleoside analog family of drugs. It works by blocking the creation of new DNA which results in cell death.

Side effects I experienced: Fatigue, hair thinning.

Xeloda (Capecitabine) – inside the body this converts to 5-Fluoruoracil through which it acts. It belongs to the family of drugs known as Fluoropyrimidines, which also includes 5-Fluorouracil and Tegafur. Taken orally in tablet form.

Side effects I experienced: Severe weight gain (moon face), severe diarrhoea, nausea, severe fatigue.

Letrozole (Aromatase Inhibitor) - experienced severe joint pain.

Dexymethadrone (steroid) – experienced insomnia, weight gain, increase in appetite.

Kytril (anti-nausea) – experienced very severe constipation.

Concor - contains Bisoprolol (which is a Beta Blocker) and is used to slow down the heart beat and manage high blood pressure.

Cordarone (Amiodarone) – antiarrhythmic medication used to treat irregular heartbeat.

Useful Cancer Patient Facebook Groups for Clear Cell specifically:

• Ovarian Cancer Clear Cell Women

• Clear Cell Renal Cell Carcinoma

Ovarian Cancer Charitable and Support Websites with lots of information:

• OCRA – Ovarian Cancer Research Alliance www.ocrahope.org also has a Facebook site

• Ovacome a UK Ovarian Cancer charity www.ovacome.org.uk also has a Facebook site

• Penny Brohn a UK Charity supporting all types of women's cancer www.pennybrohn.org.uk also has a Facebook site

• Target Ovarian Cancer

www.targetovariancancer.org.uk also has a Facebook site

• Not Ovarian Cancer specific but for English speaking women with cancer in Hong Kong – my support group Cancer Connect which has a Facebook group

Cookery Books I find useful:

NOURISH, The Cancer Care Cookbook by Christine Bailey (Penny Brohn Cancer Care)

The Rainbow Diet by Chris Woollams

The Clever Guts Diet Recipe Book by Dr Claire Bailey

How To Eat Better by James Wong

Great British Soups by New Covent Garden Soup Co.

Blended Soups by Elsa Petersen-Schepelern

The Anti-Inflammatory Cookbook by Jasmine King

Reference books I find useful:

Curing Cancer with immunotherapy by Rene Chee PHD and Edward Chee MS

The Cancer Revolution by Patricia Peat

How to Beat Cancer by Chris Woollams

Vital Strategies in Cancer by Dr Jim Roach

Managing Mould by Sarah Rigby

How to Starve Cancer by Jane McLelland

The Immunotherapy Revolution by Dr Jason Williams MD, DABR

Other useful websites:

Memorial Sloane Kettering – 'About Herbs', botanicals and other products www.mskcc.org

Explains the interactions between herbs etc with cancer drugs, plus their uses and side effects. Also has an app but for iPhone only.

www.nccn.org for clinical research and evidence also has an app

www.ncbi.nim.nih.gov for clinical research and evidence

www.iherb.com great site for ordering good value supplements, delivered by Santa Fe with free shipping if spending over HK$300. Also has an app

https://m.scmp.com.lifestyle.article One Women's Hong Kong Ovarian Cancer Journey and her positive message for fellow sufferers, their friends and family (my article in the 'South China Morning Post') and there is an updated one also to launch the book

Fundraising:

It is always better to get your friends to do fundraising events for you, as they can also then get their friends involved to sponsor them or support them, that way you can reach a wider network of people.

Donations are good and I am so grateful for all of mine, but they only come from one person.

Ideas that my dear wonderful friends have used and also things that we have done:

• For an occasion like Christmas - hold a Christmas fair with a raffle, make chocolates or chutney, hold a carol singing event.

• Do a sponsored tandem paraglide, sponsored cycle ride, sponsored run, sponsored sky dive.

• Have someone shave their head or dye their hair a wacky colour. Shave off a beard or moustache that you've had for years.

• Get friends to donate clothes to sell online – we made HK$8,000 (£800) doing this, or hold a SWISH event with clothes donations.

• As dogs are big here I made dog treats, peanut or pumpkin flavour.

• One friend organised a junk trip together with an onboard auction, with the kind support of her company and clients and raised HK$100,000 (£10,000).

Be creative! Friends and family really want to help. I can't thank all mine enough for all the fundraising and donations they did to get me my first 5 immunotherapy treatments.

Dealing with Insurance Companies:

This is truly never easy, but we need them for our treatment if you are in a country that uses a private medical system. My insurance supplied by my company, is for sure, keeping me alive, as without it I wouldn't be able to afford my treatments. That's a fact!

Things to note:

• Firstly know your insurance policy, what it covers and its limits.

• Get all the contacts of the people you need to know. i.e. The Claims Department, The Medical Team for pre-approving treatment costs. A Case Manager, if there is one, that you can go to in an emergency. Or, for my insurance, I have a Members e-mail address, which gets a much quicker response than the others.

• If you need to get cover quickly, say you are in pain and they will react very fast!

• All cover has to be medically necessary, so ensure that you have all your reports handy when making a claim i.e. Completed insurance claim form, receipt for treatment, any relevant reports or referral letters from your surgeon or oncologist. Insurance companies like their paperwork!

• Most clinics or hospitals will take a Guarantee of Payment. So if you are having long term treatment in a clinic or hospital then ask about setting up a Guarantee of Payment.

• Try to get treated in a hospital that does direct billing for your specific insurance company. It's so much easier if you are for instance having surgery, and the costs run over your GOP, the hospital can then contact the insurance company directly.

• Get approval for anything over the minimum claim limit to be sure it will be reimbursed to you. I have a limit of US$500. So anything that costs over that I need to get pre-approval.

• If you get approval refused for a treatment which you think you should have covered, get your oncologist involved and appeal, don't just accept no. I appealed on my first NG Sequencing test, as it was deemed an experimental test at the time and got this covered. The other later 2 weren't covered either and my appeal was refused but I figured getting one covered was good!

Clinical Research and Articles:

(Many have other references listed at the end of the article which the author has drawn information from, so do read these also, many of which are free to read on sites like Pub Med)

<u>Endometriosis relationship to Clear Cell Ovarian Cancer:</u>

• Pearce CL, Templeton C, Rossing MA et all

Association between endometriosis and risk of histological subtypes of ovarian cancer: a pooled analysis of case control studies (Lancet Oncol 2012)

• Kim HS, Kim TH, Chung HH et al......

Risk and Prognosis of OC in women with endometriosis: a meta-analysis (British Cancer Journal 2014, 10: 1878 – 1890)

<u>Clear Cell Ovarian Cancer resistance to platinum based drugs:</u>

• Changshuai Lyu, Yinglan Zhang and Jinghe Lang, Xingnan Zhou

Arid1a gene silencing reduces the sensitivity of OCCC to Cisplatin (Exp Ther Med 2016 2nd November)

Similarity Between Clear Cell Ovarian Cancer and Clear Cell Renal Cancer:

• Jennifer Xji, Yi Kan Wang, Dawn R Cochrane and David G Huntsman

Clear cell carcinomas of the ovary and kidney: clarity through genomics (The Journal of Pathology volume 244, issue 5, 17th Jan 2018)

Cannabis Interactions with Immunotherapy:

• James Nam, Pharm D

Cannabis reduces response rate to immunotherapy for cancer (Oncology Nurse Advisor, Sept 2017)

Obesity linked to Immunotherapy :

• Fran Lowry

Paradox: Obesity promotes tumours but boosts immunotherapy (Medscape medical oncology news 28th Nov 2018) NB: clinically unproven commentary

KRAS gene resistance to radiotherapy:

• Meng Wang, Jing Han and Henning Willers

Radiation resistance in KRAS mutated lung cancer is enabled by stem-like properties mediated by an osteo portin EGFR pathway (www.ncbi.nim.nih.gov)

SBRT effective combined with Immunotherapy:

• Ralph R. Weichselbaum, Hua Liang, Yang-Xin Fu

Radiotherapy and immunotherapy: a beneficial liaison? (Nature reviews oncology 14.365-379 2017)

• Chase Doyle

Combination radiotherapy and immunotherapy appears safe and clinically active in advanced solid tumours (25th Feb 2018 – www.ascopost.com)

Clinical trial for Pembrolizumab combined with Pazopanib:

• Simon Chowdhury, David F. McDermott, Martin Henner Voss, Robert E. Hawkins, Paola Aimone, Maurizio Voi, Naeije Isabelle, Yi Wu and Jeffrey R. Infante

A phase I/II study to assess the safety and efficacy of pazopanib and pembrolizumab in patients with advanced renal cell carcinoma (Journal of Clinical Oncology ASCO 2017)

Relationship between Prolactin and KRAS genome:

• Bipin Kumar Sethi, G.V. Chanukya and V. Sri Nagesh

Prolactin and cancer: Has the orphan finally found a home? (Indian Journal of Endocrinology and Metabolism Dec 2012, supplement 2, S195-S198)

Lack of survival benefit of adjuvant chemotherapy in stage 1 clear cell ovarian cancer:

• Dave Levitan

No survival benefit with adjuvant chemotherapy for most endometrioid, ovarian clear cell cancers (Cancer Network 9th October 2017)

• Kristin Jenkins

More Chemo May Not Equal Better Outcomes in Ovarian Cancer – recurrence, survival acceptable with 3 cycles in clear cell carcinoma (Med Page today 16th January 2017)

Zejula efficacy in Non-BRCA genetic Ovarian Cancer Patients:

• The Nova Trial – www.zejula.com

<u>Clear Cell Ovarian Cancer causes Blood Clots:</u>

• Matsura Y, Robertson G, Marsden DE, Kim SN, Gebski V, Hacker NE

Thromboembolic Complications in Patients with Clear Cell Carcinoma of the Ovary (Gynecol Oncol 2007 Feb 104(2), 406-10)

<u>The Patriot Trial</u>

• M.T. Dillon, Z.Boylan, D.Smith, J.Guevara, K. Mohammed, C.Peckitt, M.Saunders, V.Banerji, G.Clack, S.A. Smith, J.F.Spicer, M.D.Forster, K.J. Kerrington

PATRIOT: A phase 1 study to assess the tolerability, safety and biological effects of a specific ataxia telangiectasia and Rad 3- related (ATR) inhibitor (AZD6738) as a single agent and in combination with palliative radiotherapy in patients with solid tumours (Clinical and Translational Radiation Oncology June 2018)

<u>The Atari Trial</u>

A Phase II study - Combining an ATR inhibitor (AZD6738) in combination with Olaparib a PARP inhibitor for gynaecological cancers with ARID1A deficient ('loss') and 'no loss'

Chief Investigator: Dr Susana Banerjee, The Royal Marsden NHS Foundation Trust

With Thanks:

It is very difficult to know where to start with this as I have so many people to thank, I fear I might miss someone, if I do apologies in advance as I don't mean to, I appreciate every single person who has supported me through this journey.

Firstly, I must thank my family, my amazing mum, my brother and sister in law and my cousins you know who you are.

My dear friend Sara who although we don't see each other so often now, for always being there for me with sound advice and so much support and love.

Ditto for my dear school friend T for all her support since the start of this journey and for coming out to visit all this way when I know she dislikes travelling.

I know she doesn't want a huge fuss but my oncologist Dr W who without her expertise I know I would not be alive today, my dear oncology nurse Tracy and the team at Chiron Clinic.

My surgeons Dr N and Professor P who without their skill I would also not be here today.

To my wonderful radiology doctor, Dr Y for his precision and knowledge in interpreting my scans.

To every single friend, family member and colleague who donated or fundraised for my initial immunotherapy treatment – too many to name but thank you from the bottom of my heart.

For my wonderful friends at Cancer Connect especially GM, CR, RL and TBL for all your continuous friendship and support.

My wonderful work colleagues and bosses for understanding PS, PH, AL, DE, PN, BS, ZW, CL, LL and SH.

To the amazing Sarah Rigby for helping me to publish this book.

For my dear friend Anne-Marie Engleman who designed the book cover despite her busy schedule and was there for me on so many tough occasions.

For Teresa and Tony who took all the stress away to manage the website and post out the books.

To the talented and amazing Quynh Lee for designing the book website.

Reader Comments:

'It's a great story. Picked it up yesterday and already on page 80. Straight up Hilary humour. Filled with good info and hope - a must read!'

'I finished your excellent book about 2 weeks ago, it's epic and incredibly inspiring. Congratulations.'

'Wow! Fuk Yu is great because it shows a person struggling with a disease, bureaucracies, political issues and remaining a human being who is kind, caring and able to have a refreshing view on life. It's truly admirable. Thank you for sharing and benefitting those struggling with a nasty disease.'

'Enjoyed reading your book, which would be very helpful to let our young doctors understand the sheer distress of being unwell.'

'Just finished your book on the flight down to Houston, MD Anderson. It's so great and I'm so glad you wrote it and published it! It will be so helpful for me. I'm not a reader and I never read books and read your book in one sitting!'

'Read the whole book last night, it's brilliant! Lots of info that I need'.

'Love your honest and open writing of your journey and the poem about your mom is beautiful. Some parts of the book made me giggle and sometimes I wanted to cry'.

'I wanted to let you know that I have just finished reading your book from cover to cover and 'enjoyed' it so much, if I can say that! I felt like I was having a conversation with you, which was so nice. Your stamina and attitude not to mention perseverance and knowledge are quite astounding. Sincere respect to you. It was/is quite moving but I had a few smiles!'

'I wanted to let you know I have started to read your book. You have been through so much I am sure this book will help others going through the process. Quite emotional reading this, it is so nice to read it though and you write as you speak which is also really nice.'

'I finished your book, and I think it will be very useful for anyone who undergoes this journey. I laughed a lot, I remembered having awful flatulence during chemo! – now I know I should have stayed near dogs and children!'

'I didn't realise the extent of the ordeal you've been through. I liked the personal observation and quips and that you didn't shy away from some of the more embarrassing side effects. The more technical aspects of the various types of treatments should be a useful reference for those with cancer and their carers.'

'The book is brilliant – I read it in a day (v unusual for me). I already know what a force of nature you are but the book just really brings that out and shows how single minded you were about not giving

up and staying alive exploring every option and that's why you're still here. How did you keep going? Just incredible.......and so helpful picked up so many useful tips and info and going to read again. Think it's a brilliant aid in terms of evaluating each stage and considering everything.'

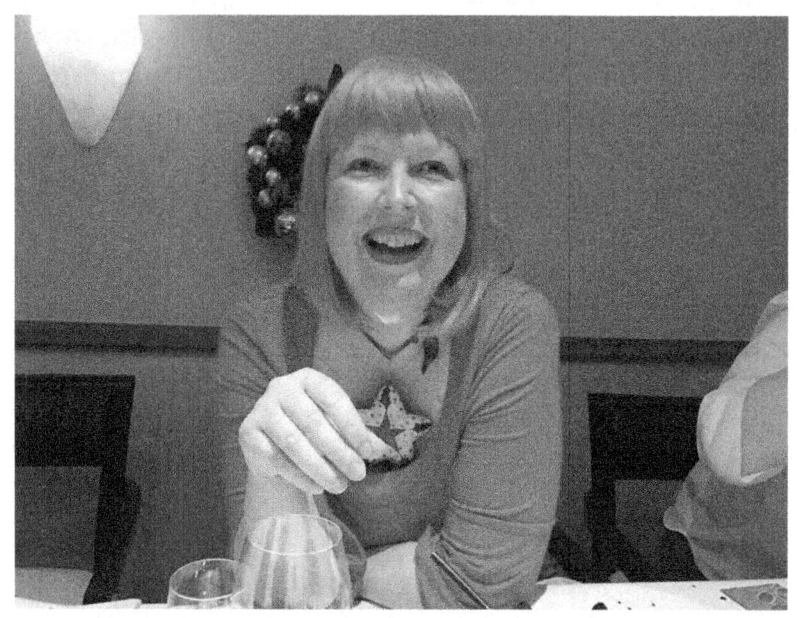

My winning outfit at the Cancer Connect Christmas dinner

(colour picture is on the book website!)

Made in United States
North Haven, CT
04 April 2024

50902216R00098